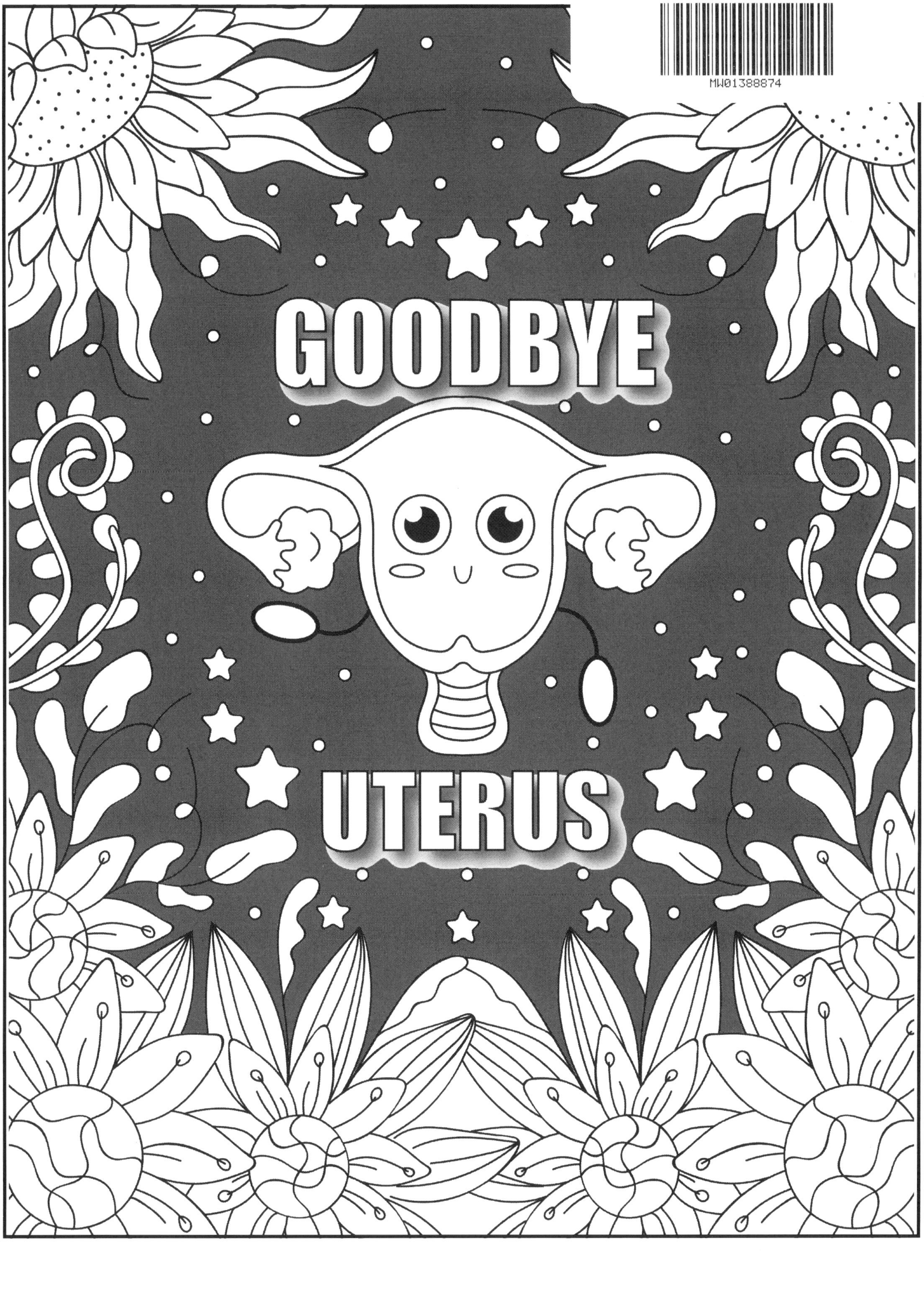
GOODBYE
UTERUS

We would like to thank you personally for purchasing this book. This activity book is a collection of 20+ funny Hysterectomy Coloring Pages, Sudoku ,Word Search and Word Scramble Puzzles.

At Sandesh Poudel Publishing we understand that having a Hysterectomy surgery can be tough. So, to let you vent out some of the stress and to help you relax we have created this activity book.

Published by Sandesh Poudel Publishing

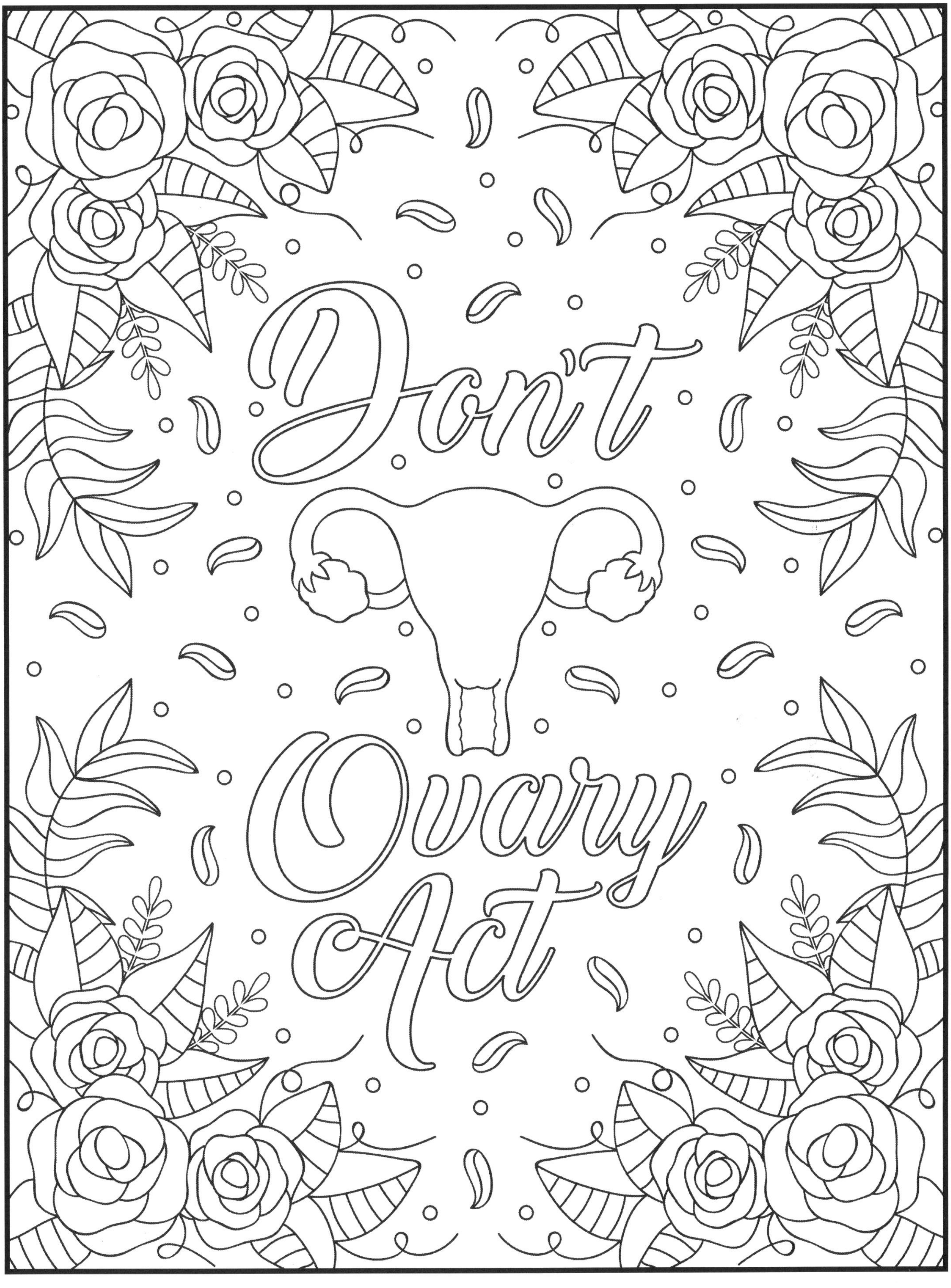
Don't
Ovary
Act

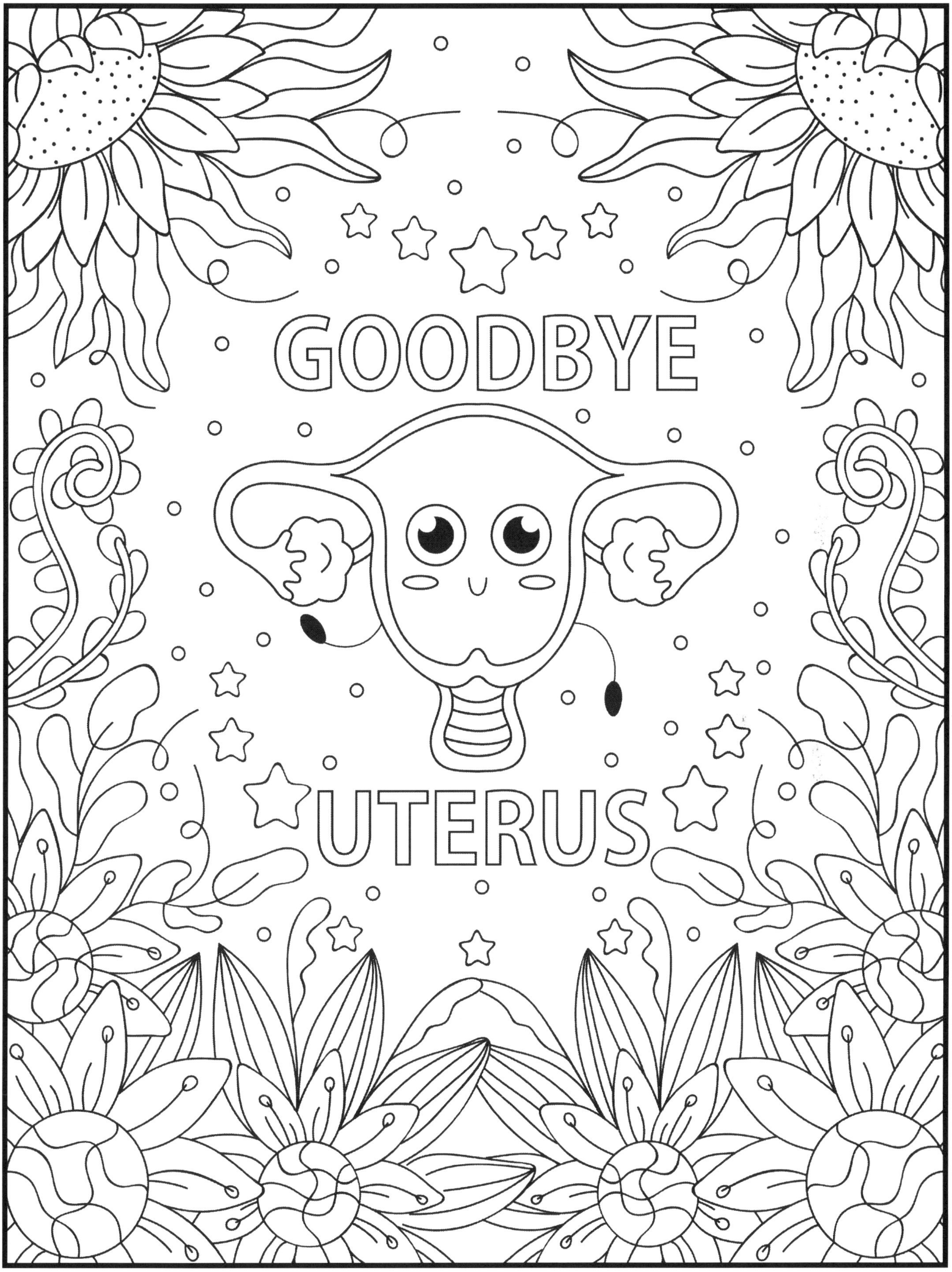
GOODBYE
UTERUS

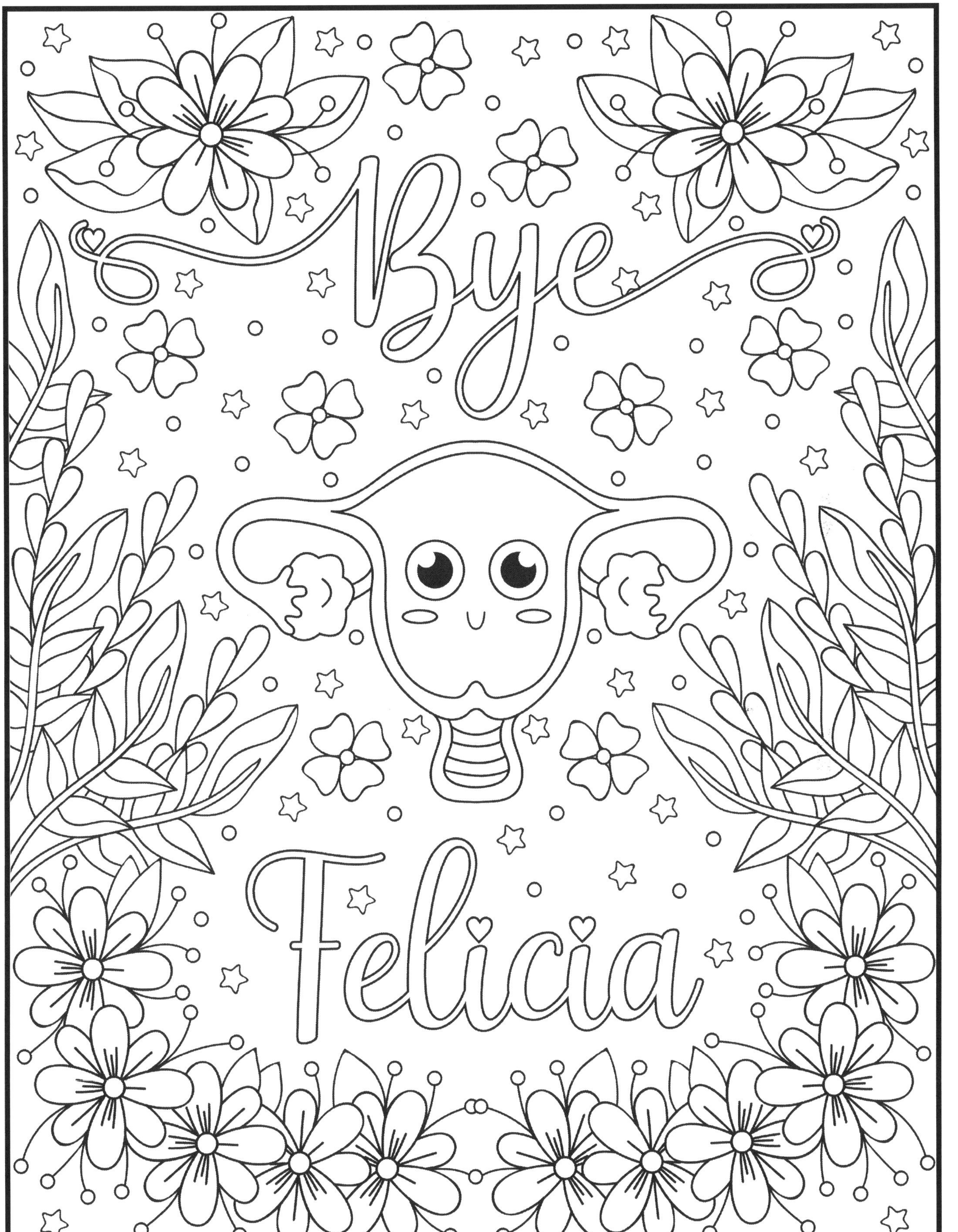
Bye
Felicia

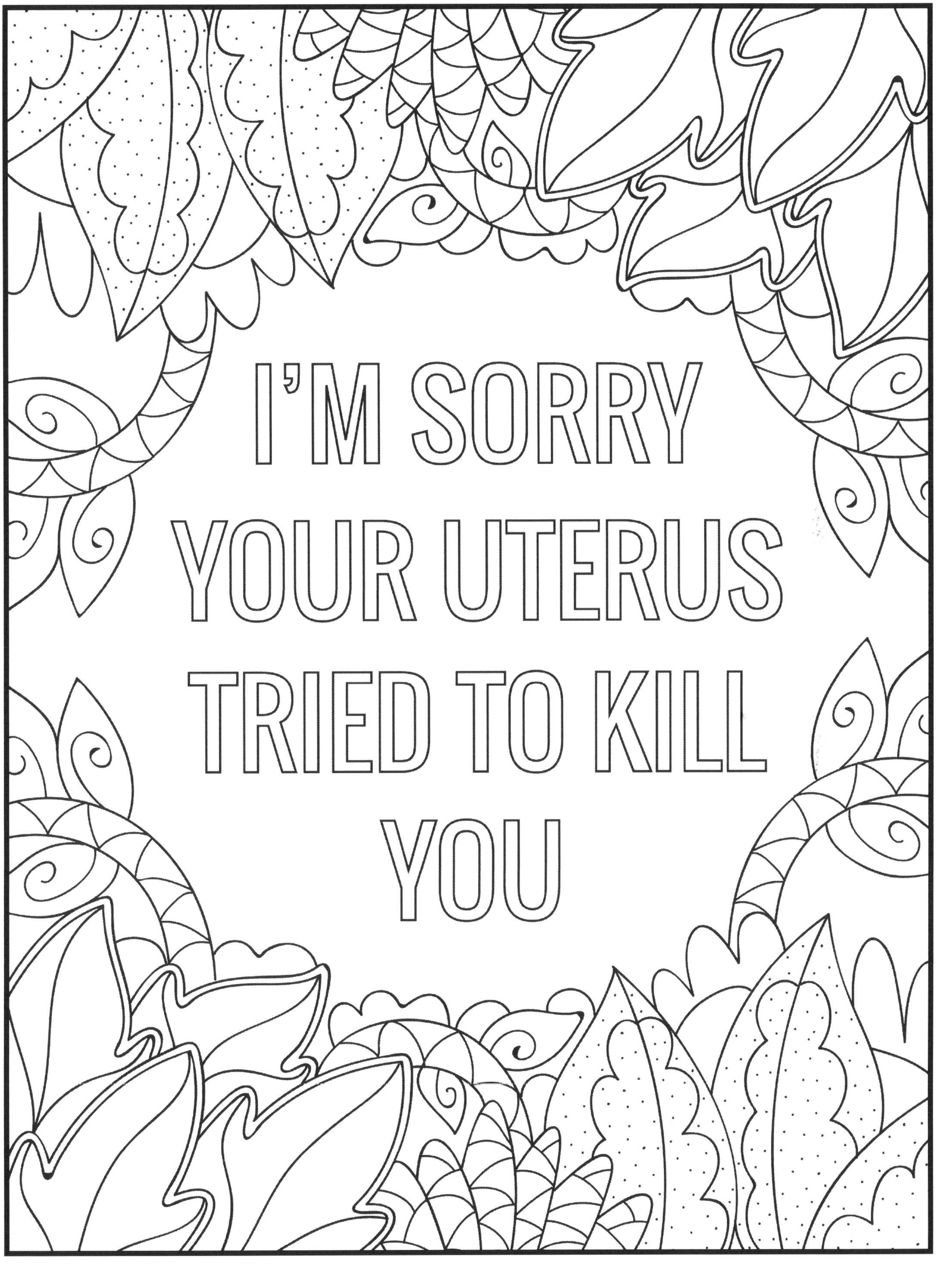
I'M SORRY
YOUR UTERUS
TRIED TO KILL
YOU

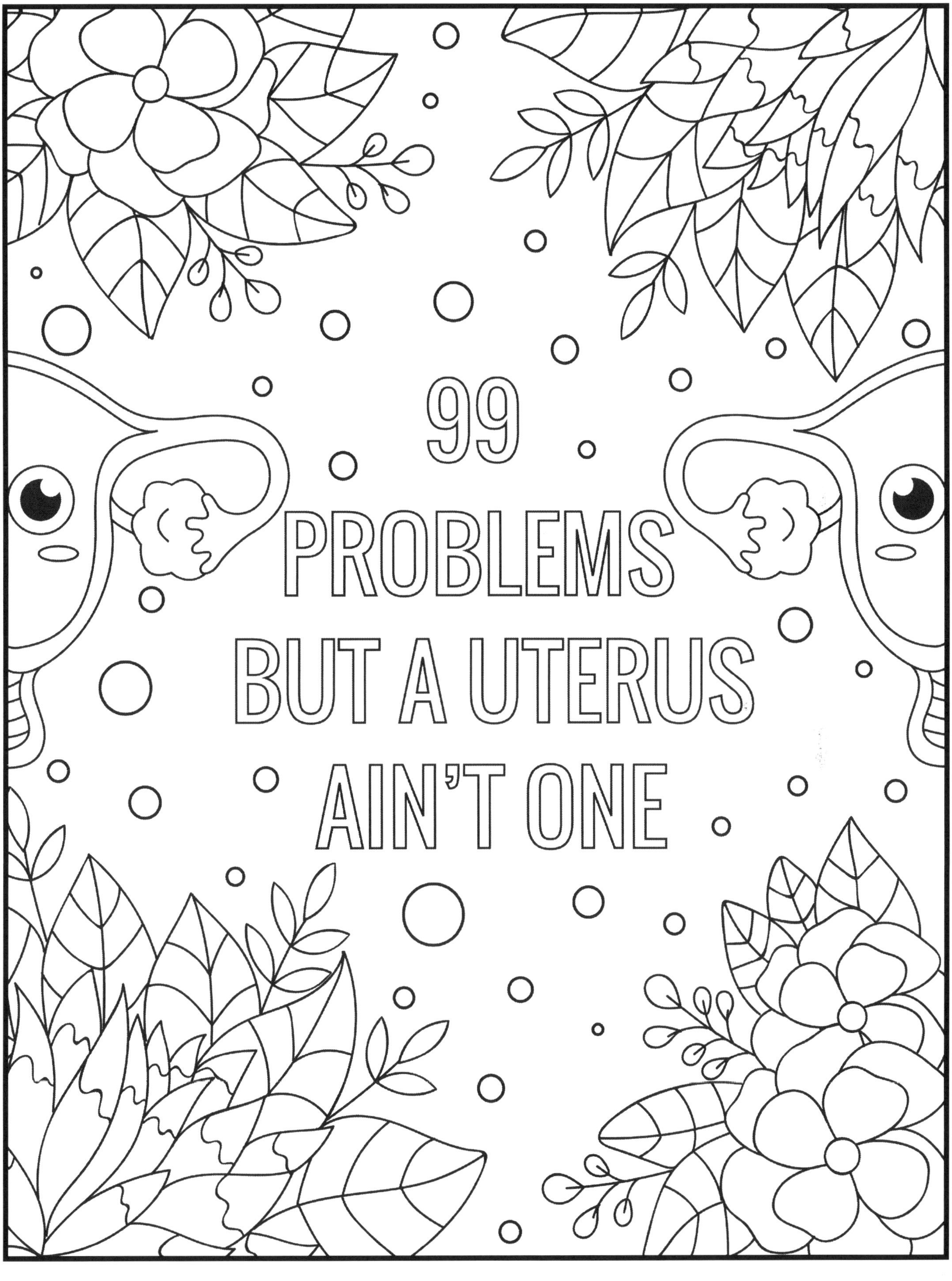
99
PROBLEMS
BUT A UTERUS
AIN'T ONE

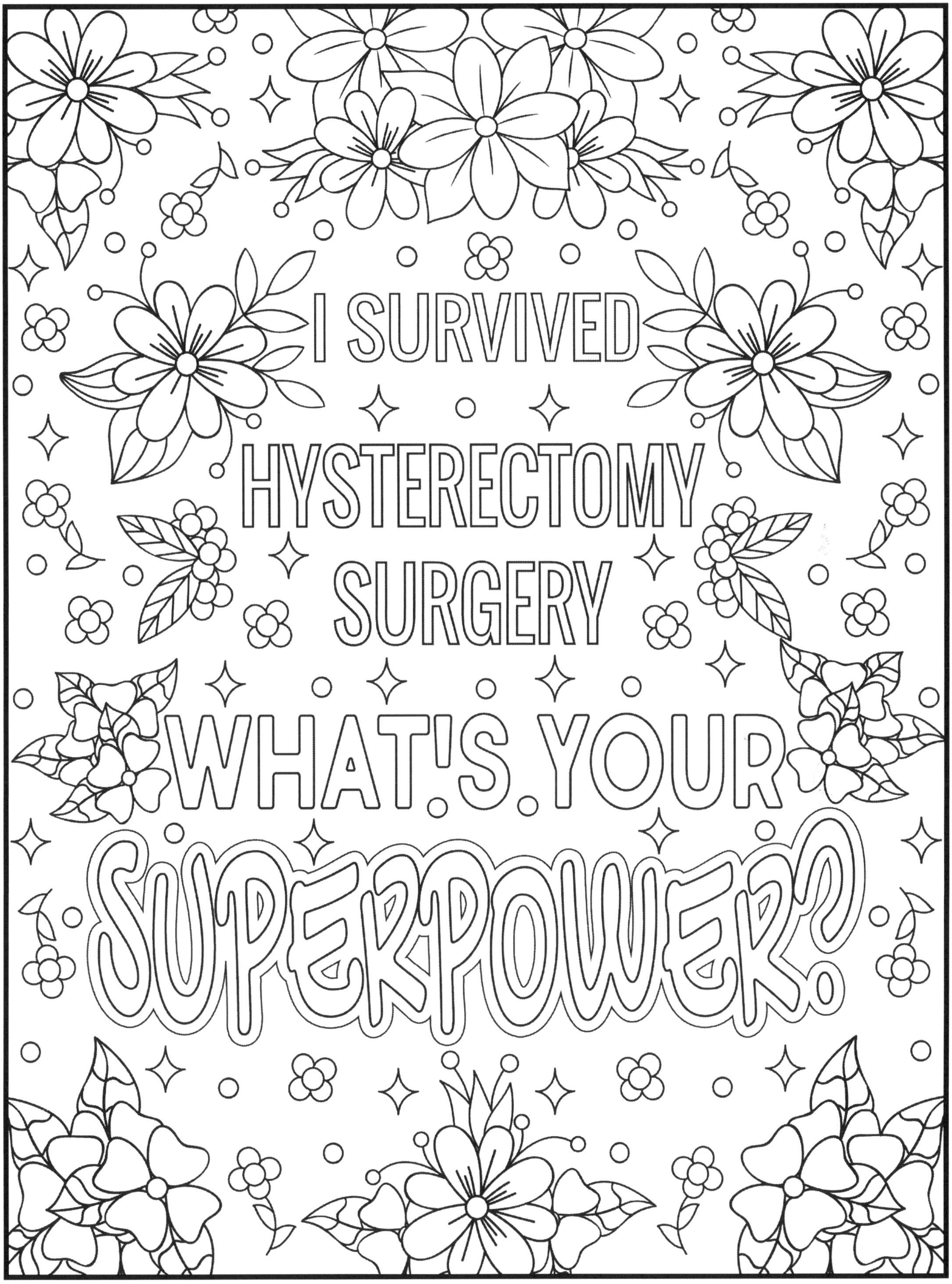
I SURVIVED
HYSTERECTOMY
SURGERY
WHAT'S YOUR
SUPERPOWER?

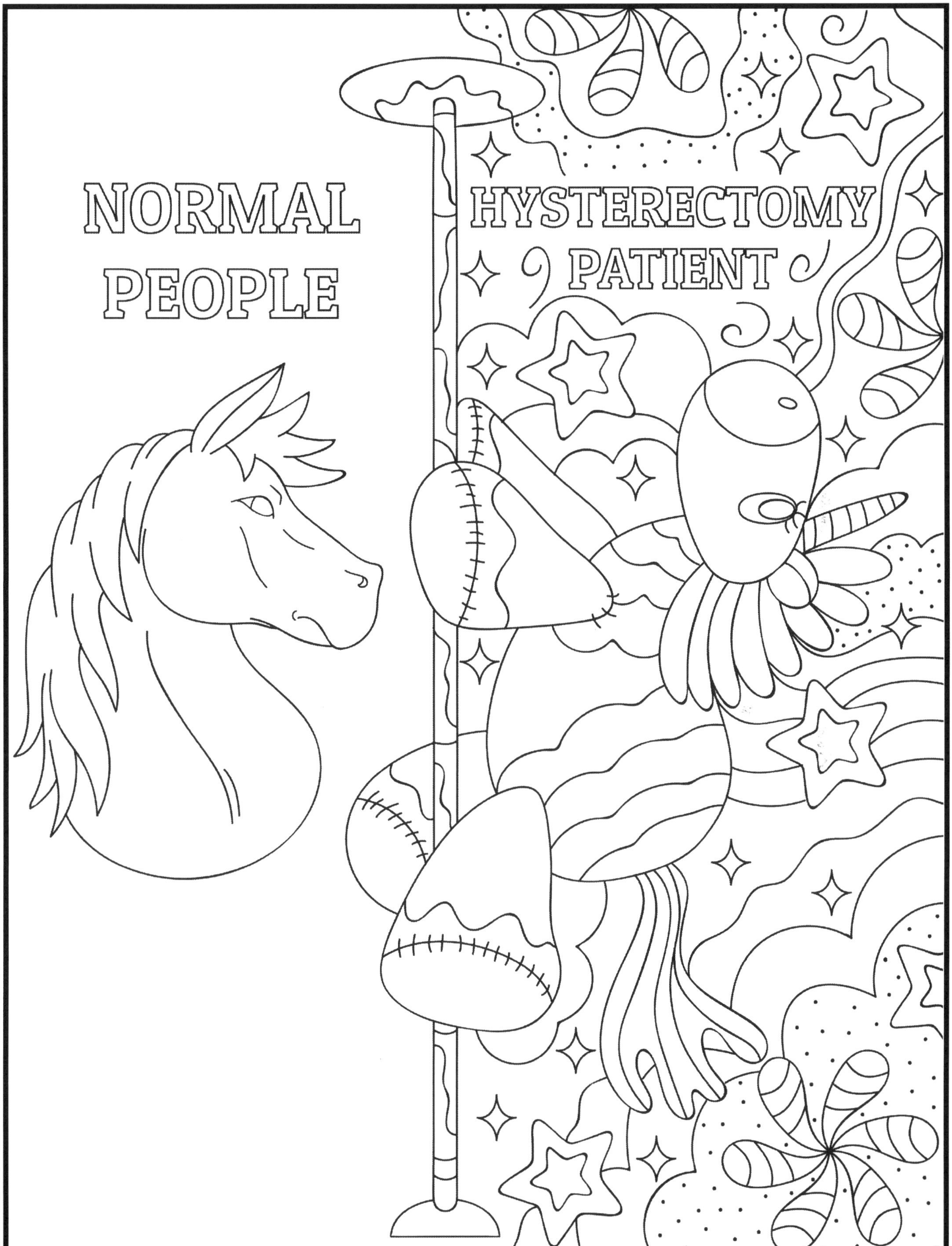
NORMAL PEOPLE
HYSTERECTOMY PATIENT

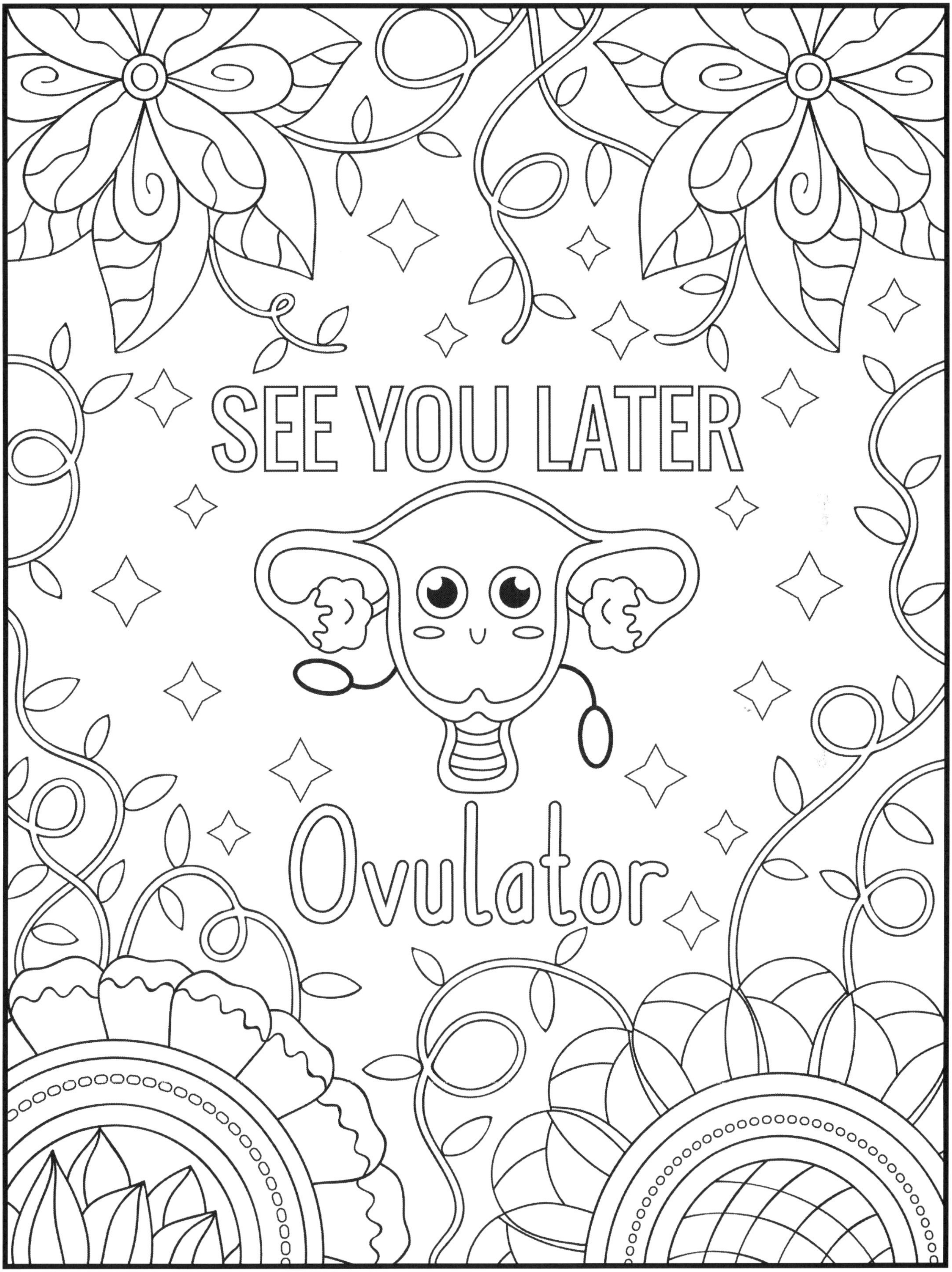
SEE YOU LATER
Ovulator

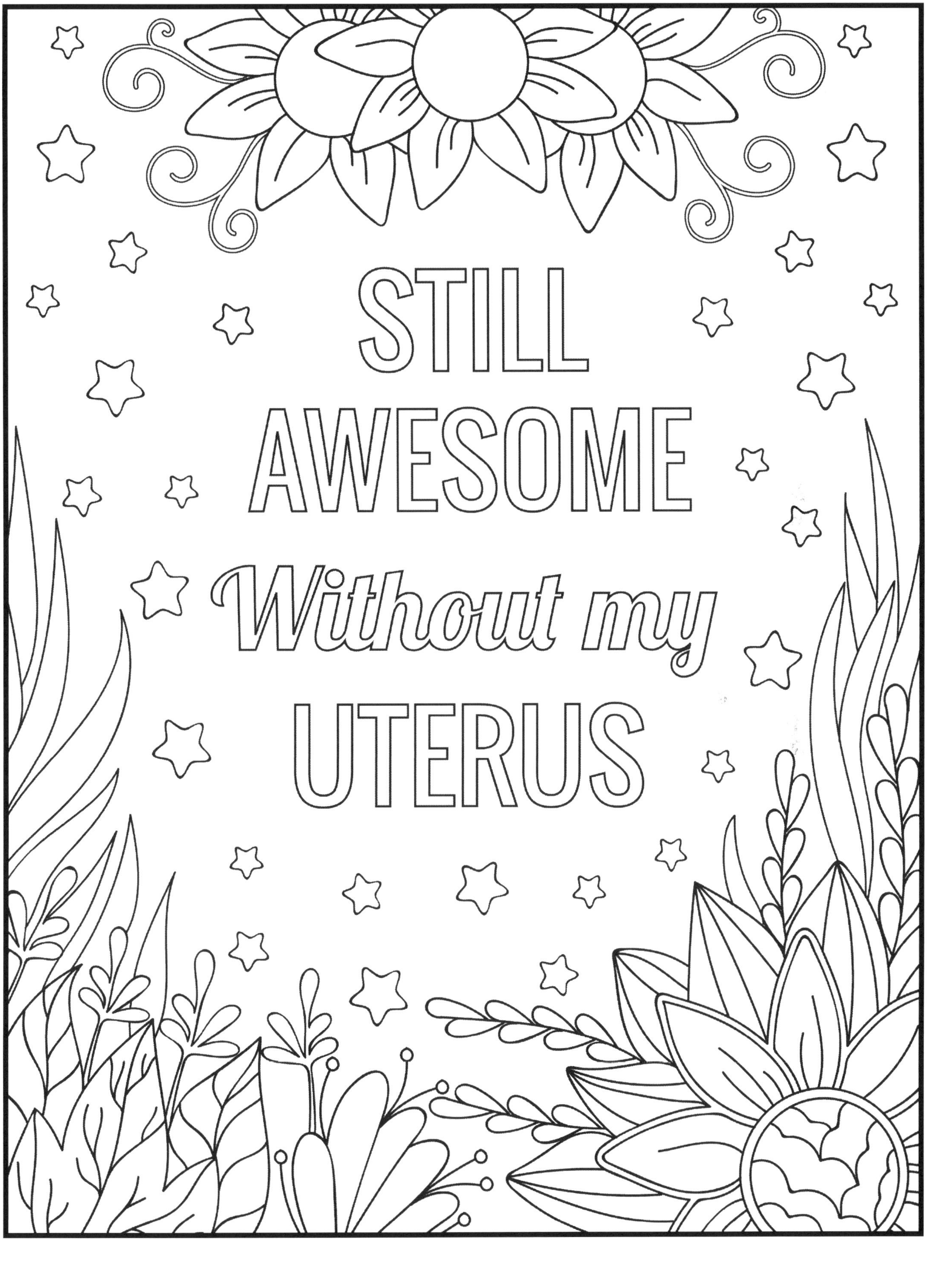
STILL
AWESOME
Without my
UTERUS

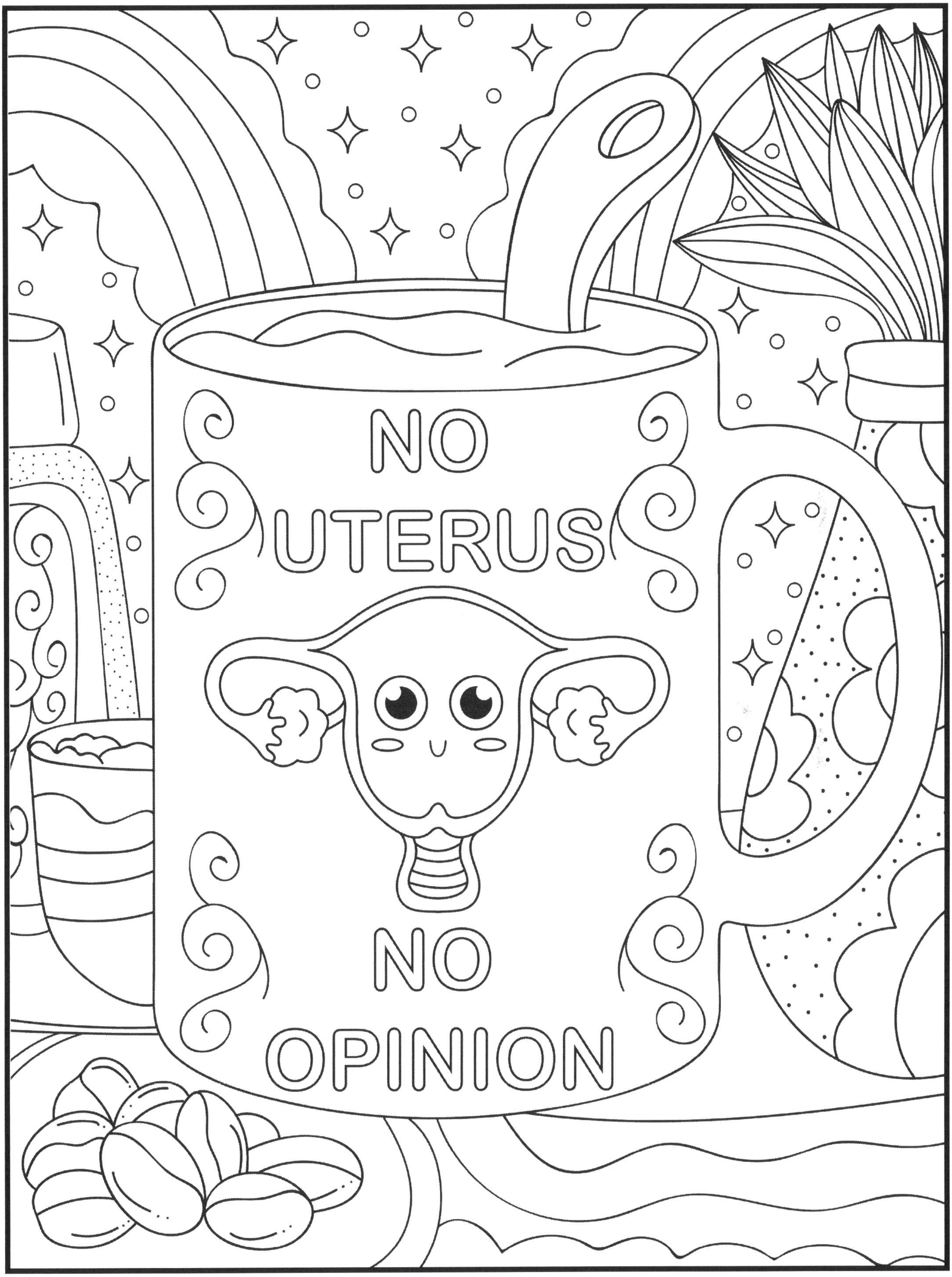
NO
UTERUS
NO
OPINION

HYSTERECTOMY

NUTRITION FACTS

AMOUNT PER SERVING: 1 GREAT SURGERY

	% DAILY VALUE*
LOVE	1000%
STRESS	0%
FRIENDS & FAMILY	1000%
HUGS & KISSES	800%
MEMORIES	600%
COURAGE	1000%

*Percentage daily values are based on your unique diet

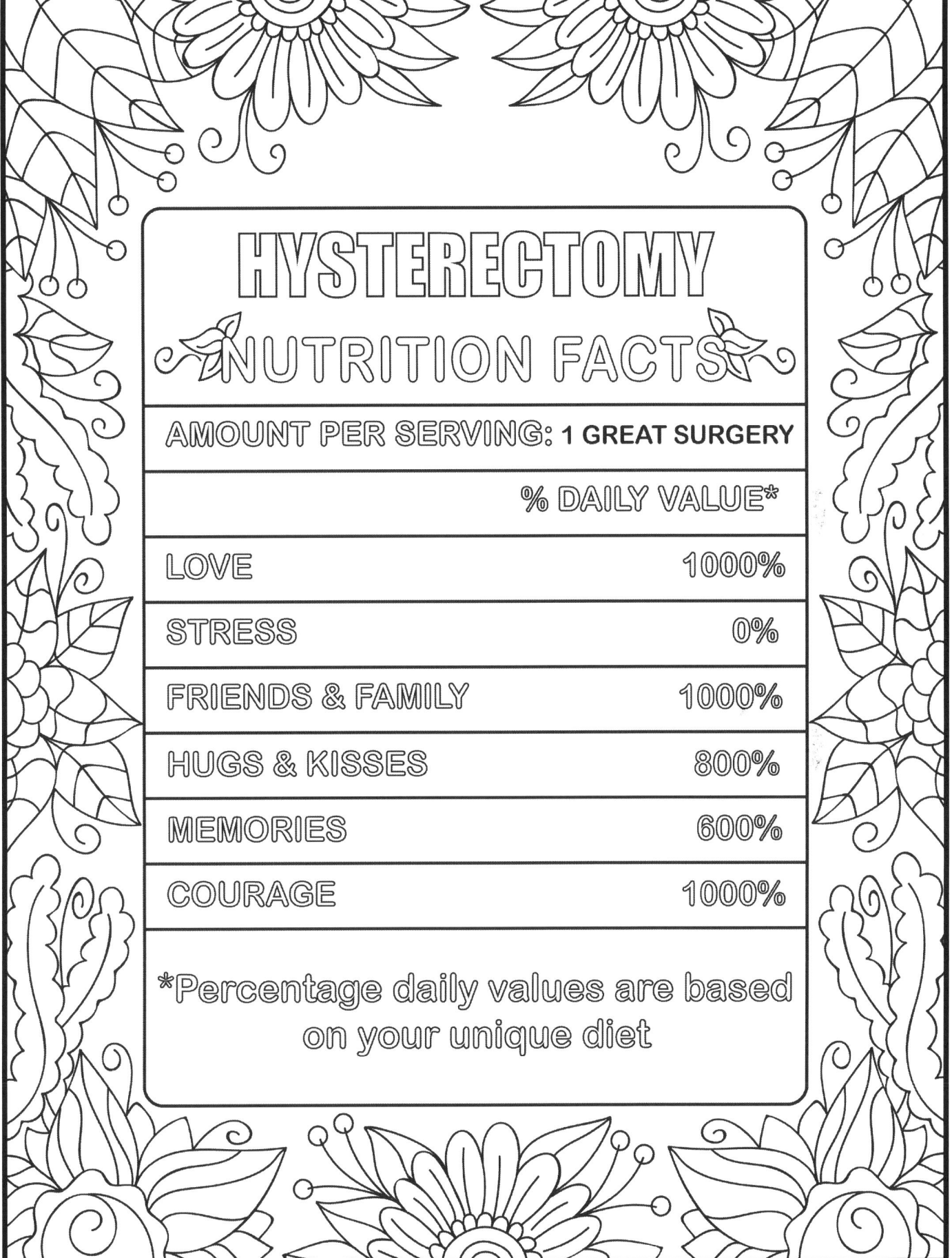

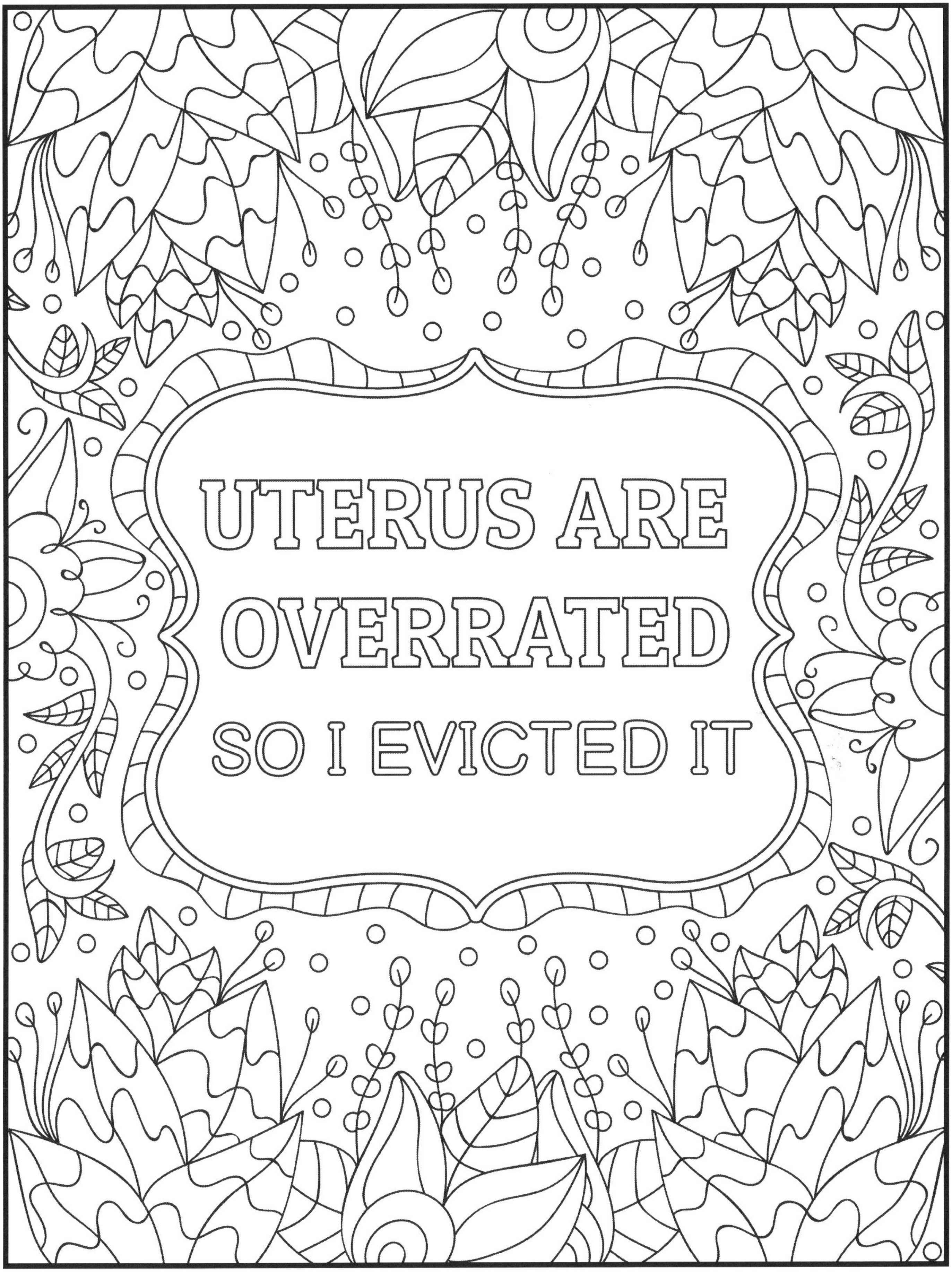
UTERUS ARE
OVERRATED
SO I EVICTED IT

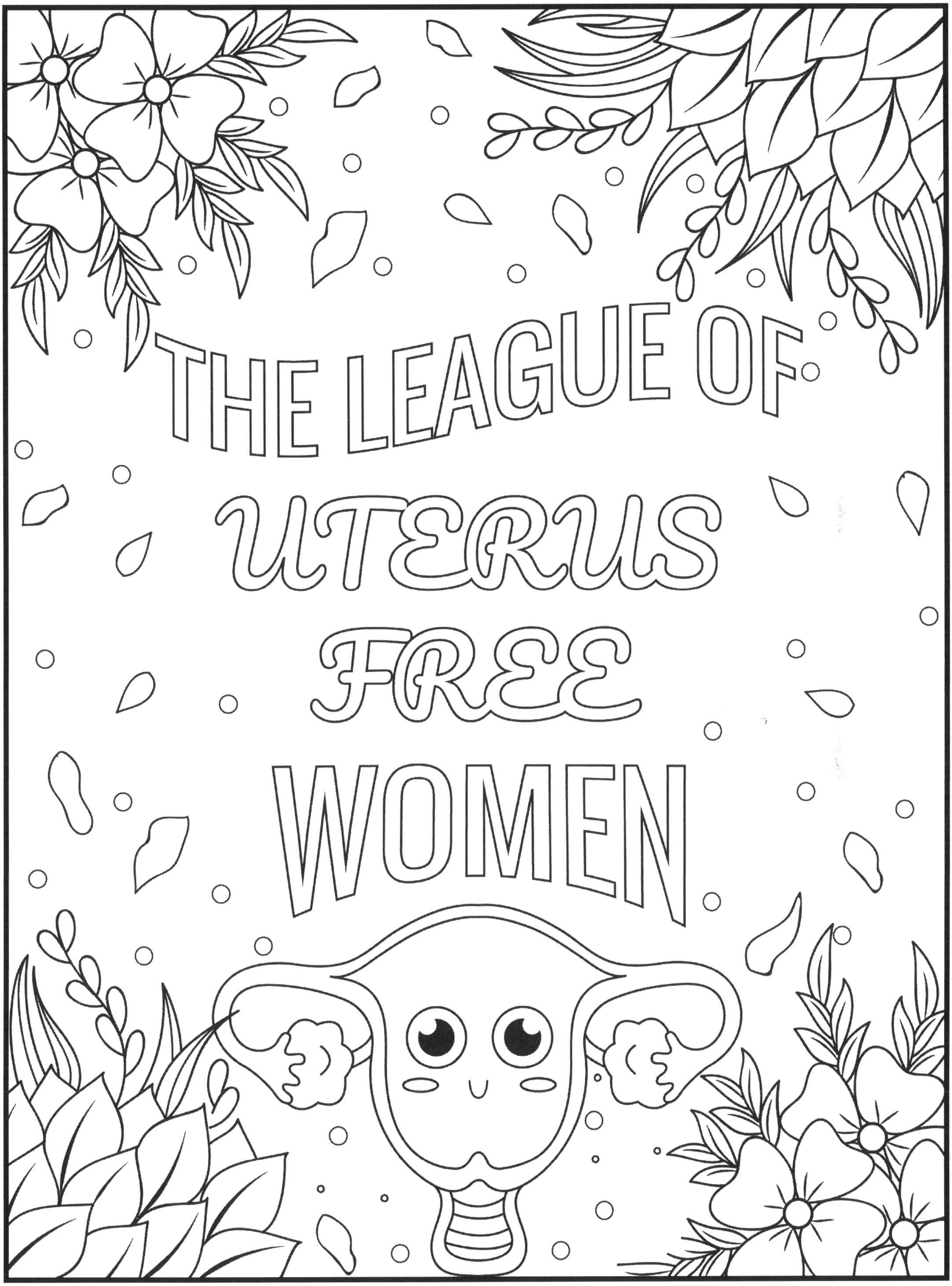
THE LEAGUE OF
UTERUS
FREE
WOMEN

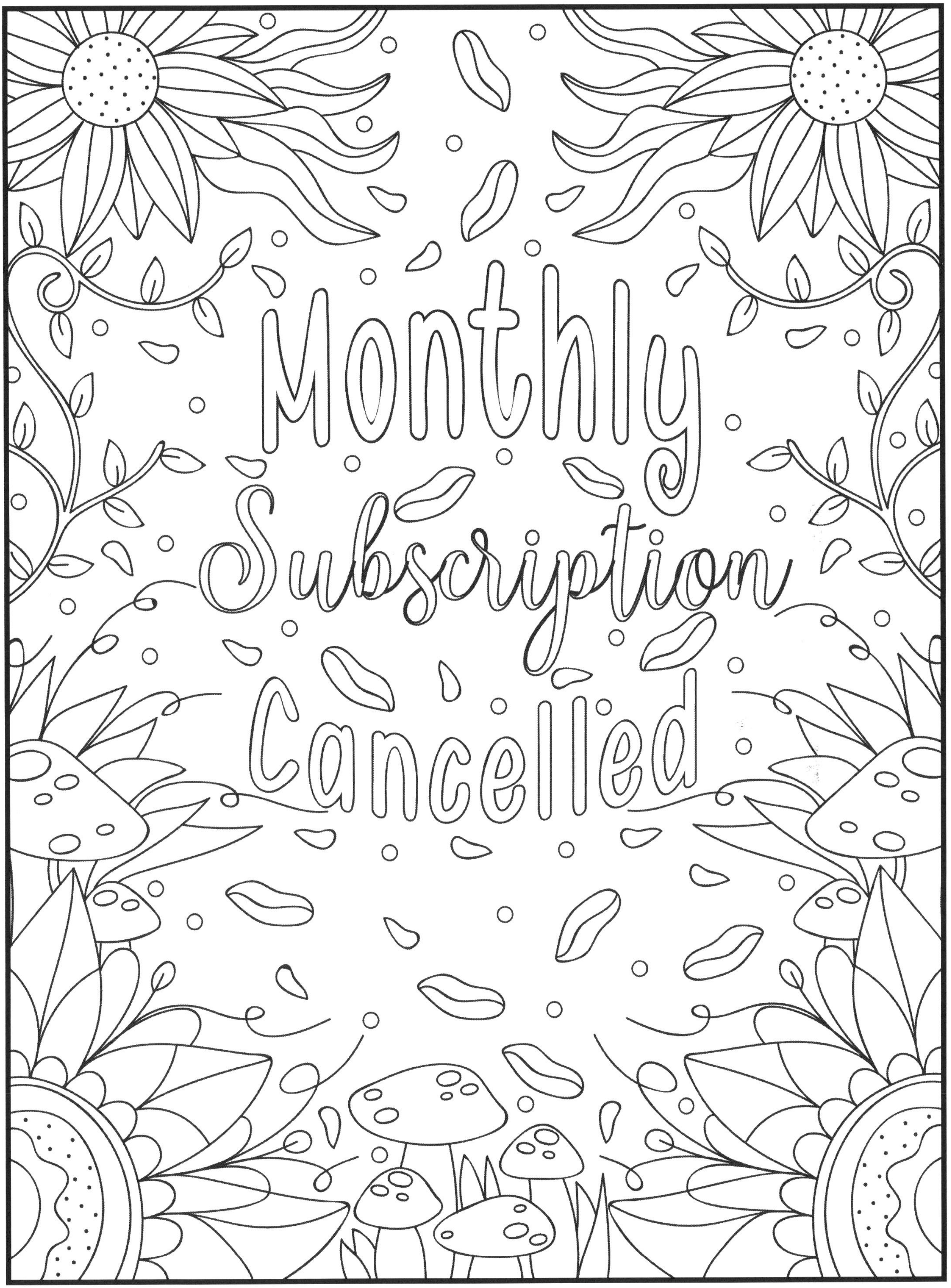
Monthly
Subscription
Cancelled

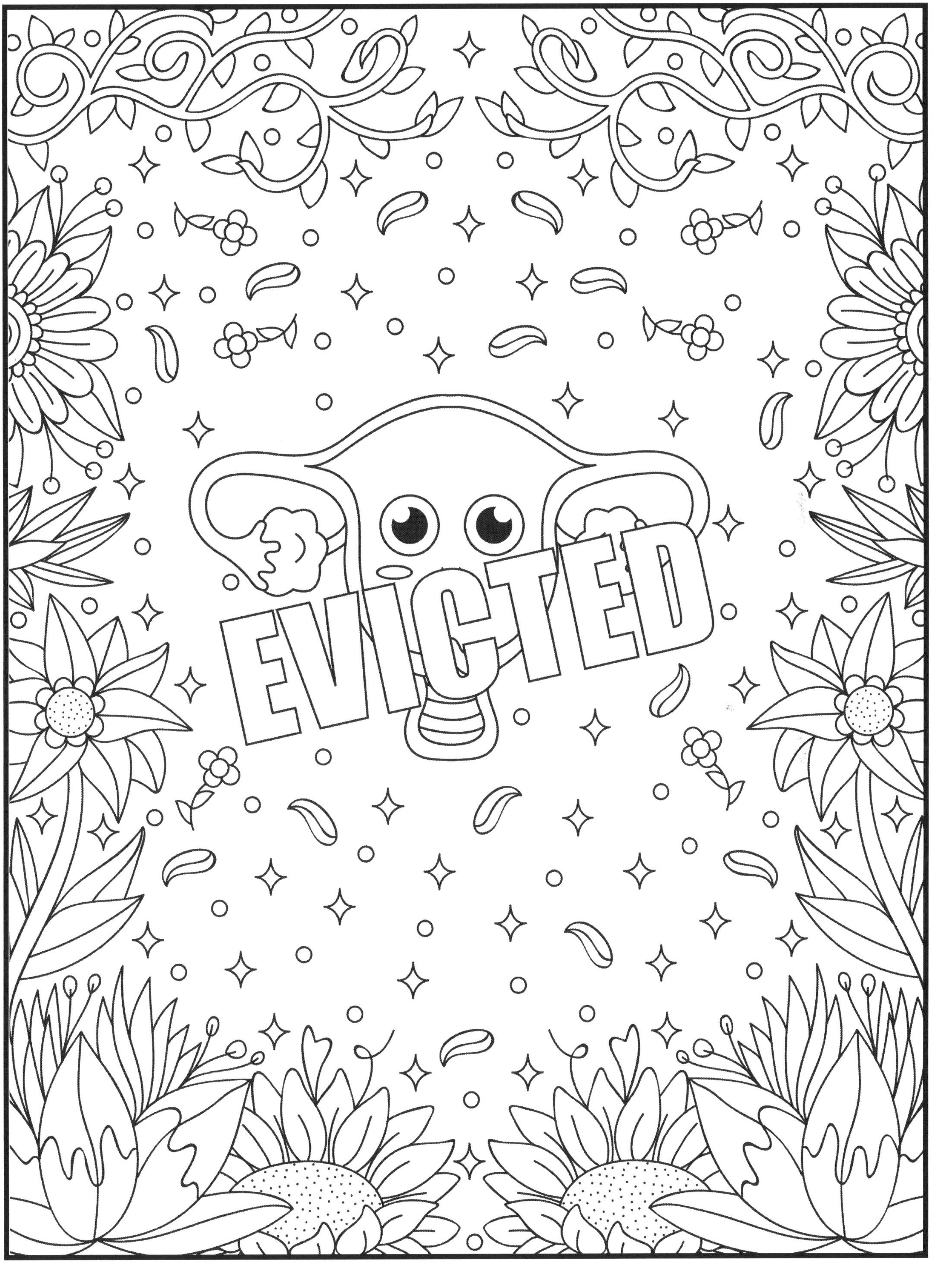
EVICTED

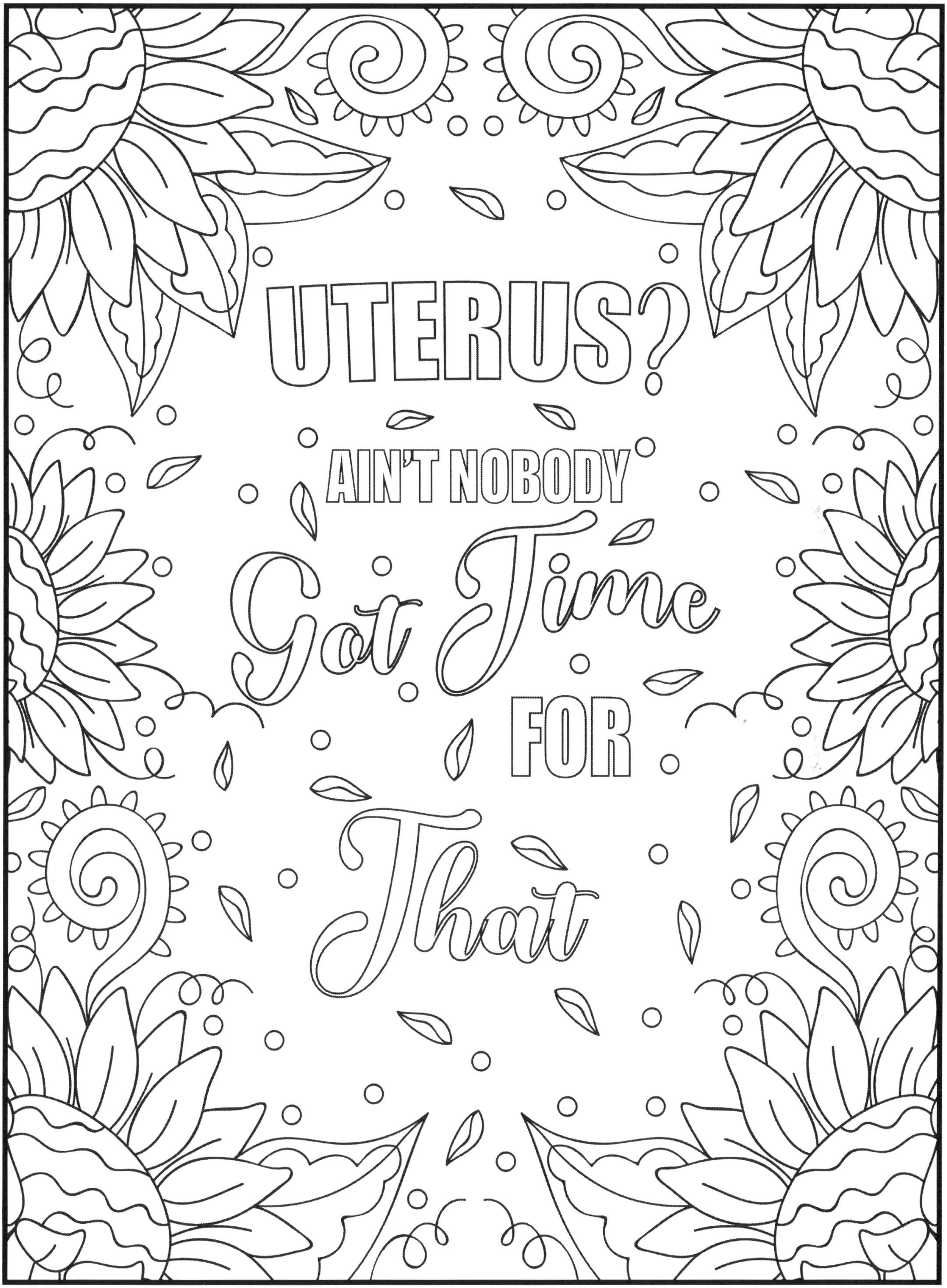
UTERUS?
AIN'T NOBODY
Got Time
FOR
That

GONE
BUT NOT
FORGOTTEN

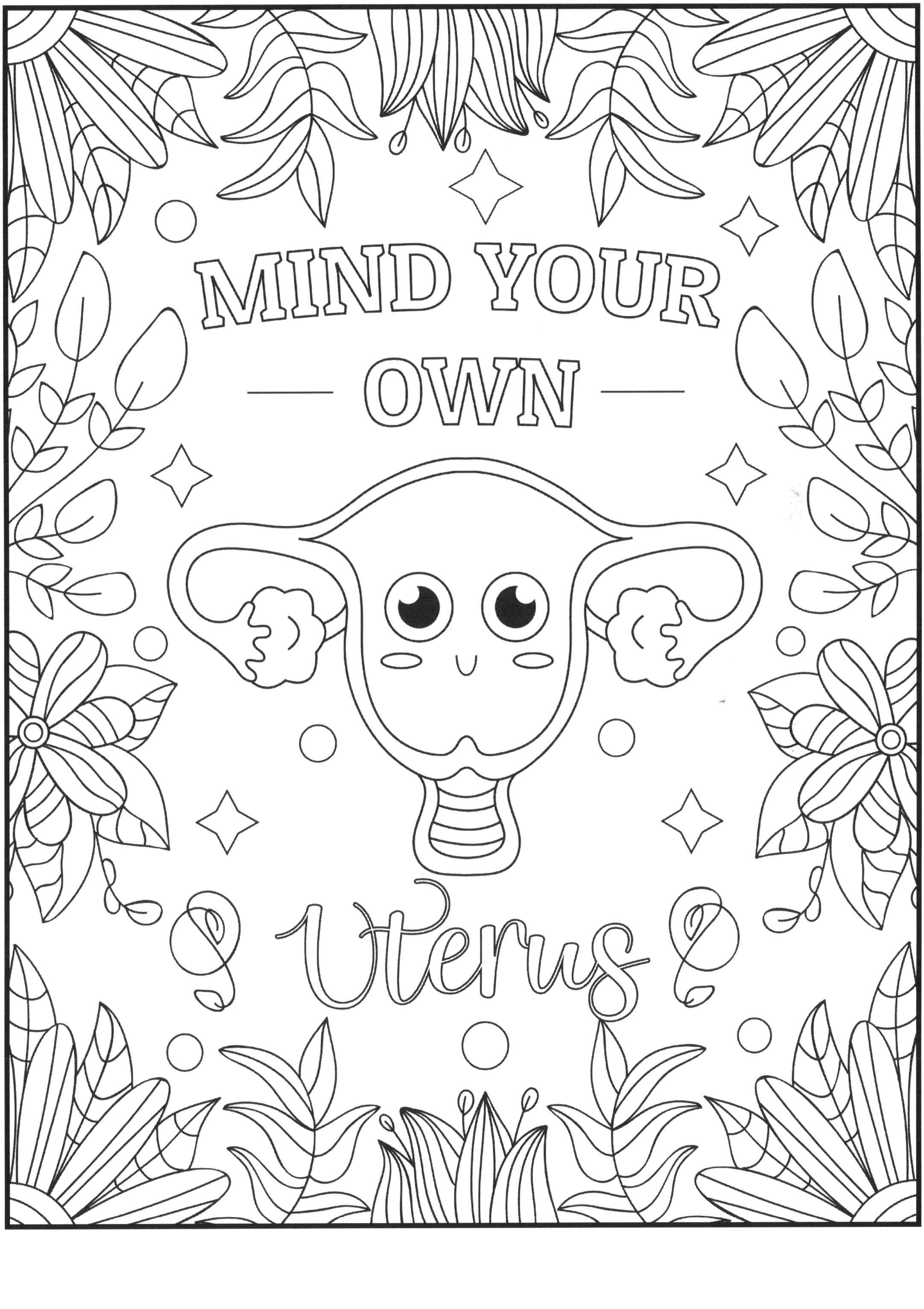
MIND YOUR
OWN
Uterus

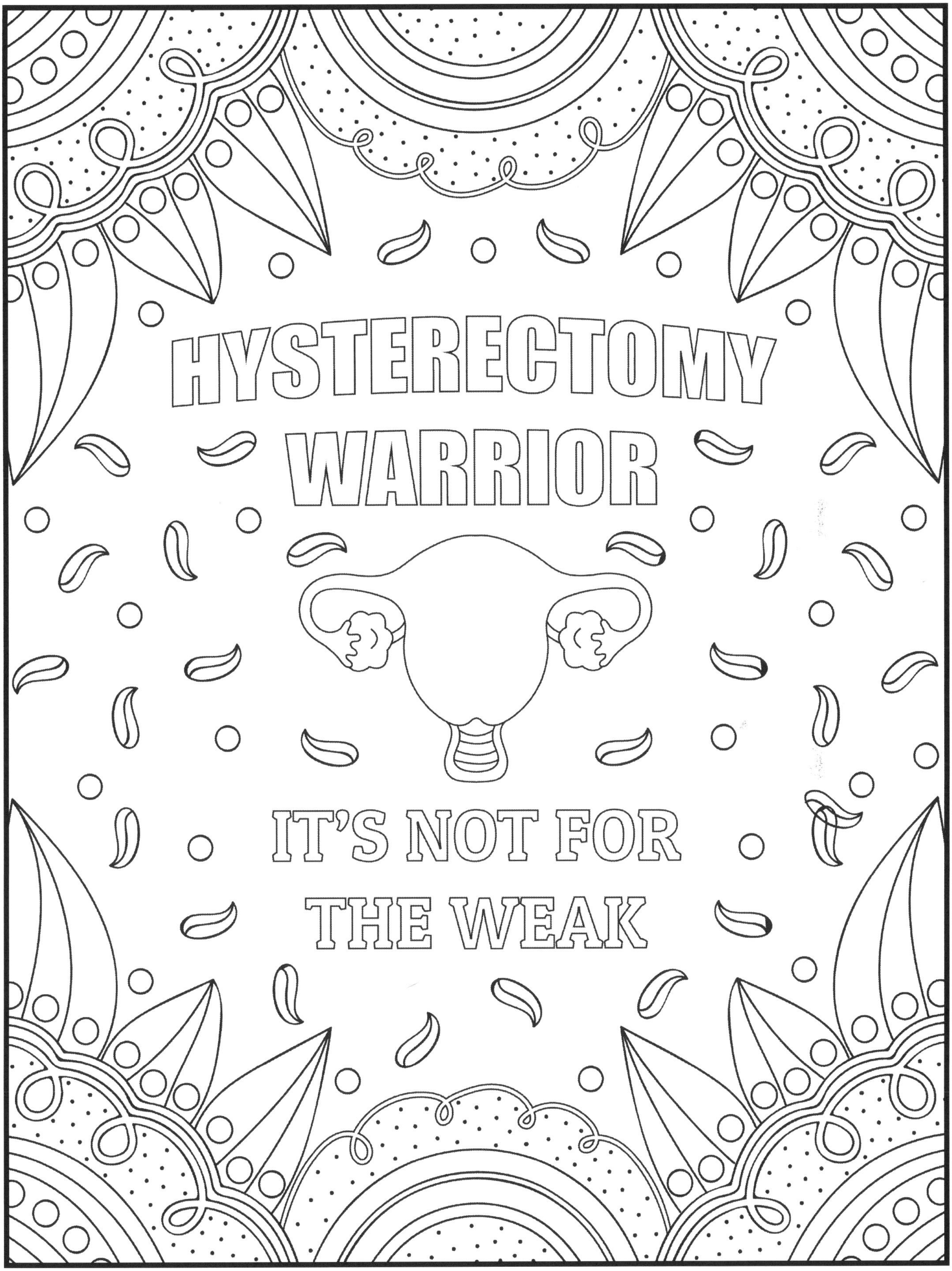
HYSTERECTOMY
WARRIOR
IT'S NOT FOR
THE WEAK

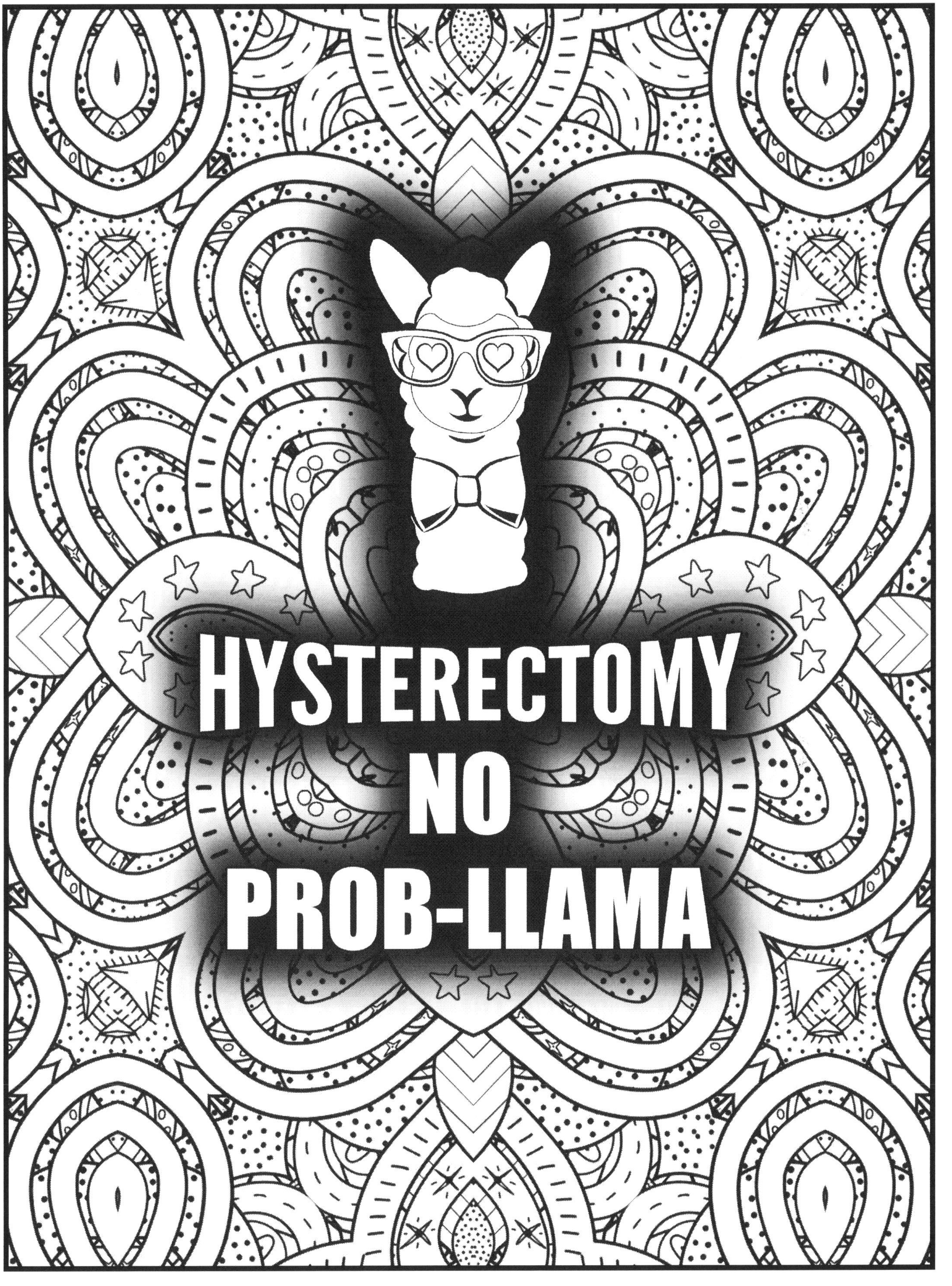
HYSTERECTOMY
NO
PROB-LLAMA

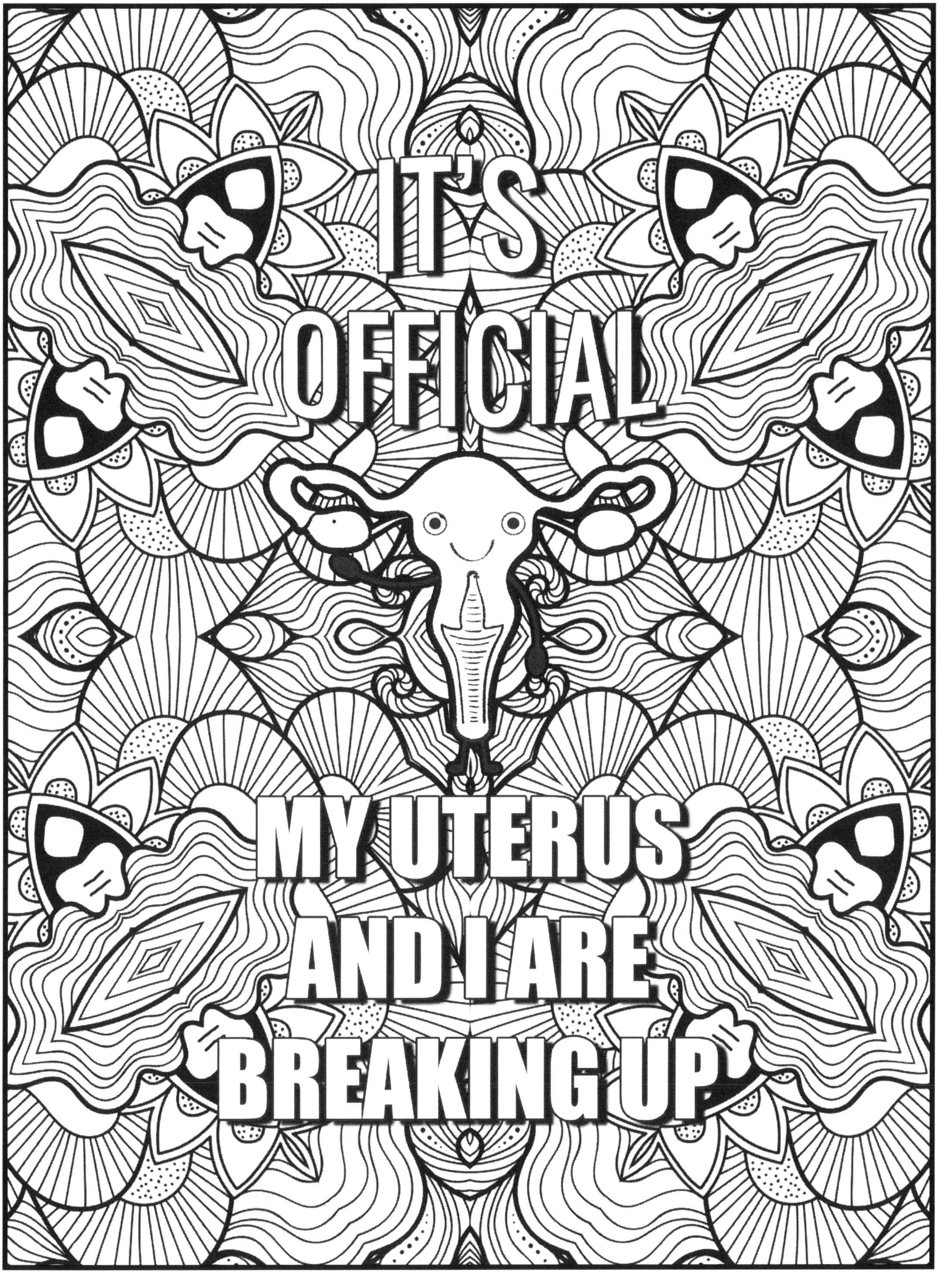
IT'S
OFFICIAL
MY UTERUS
AND I ARE
BREAKING UP

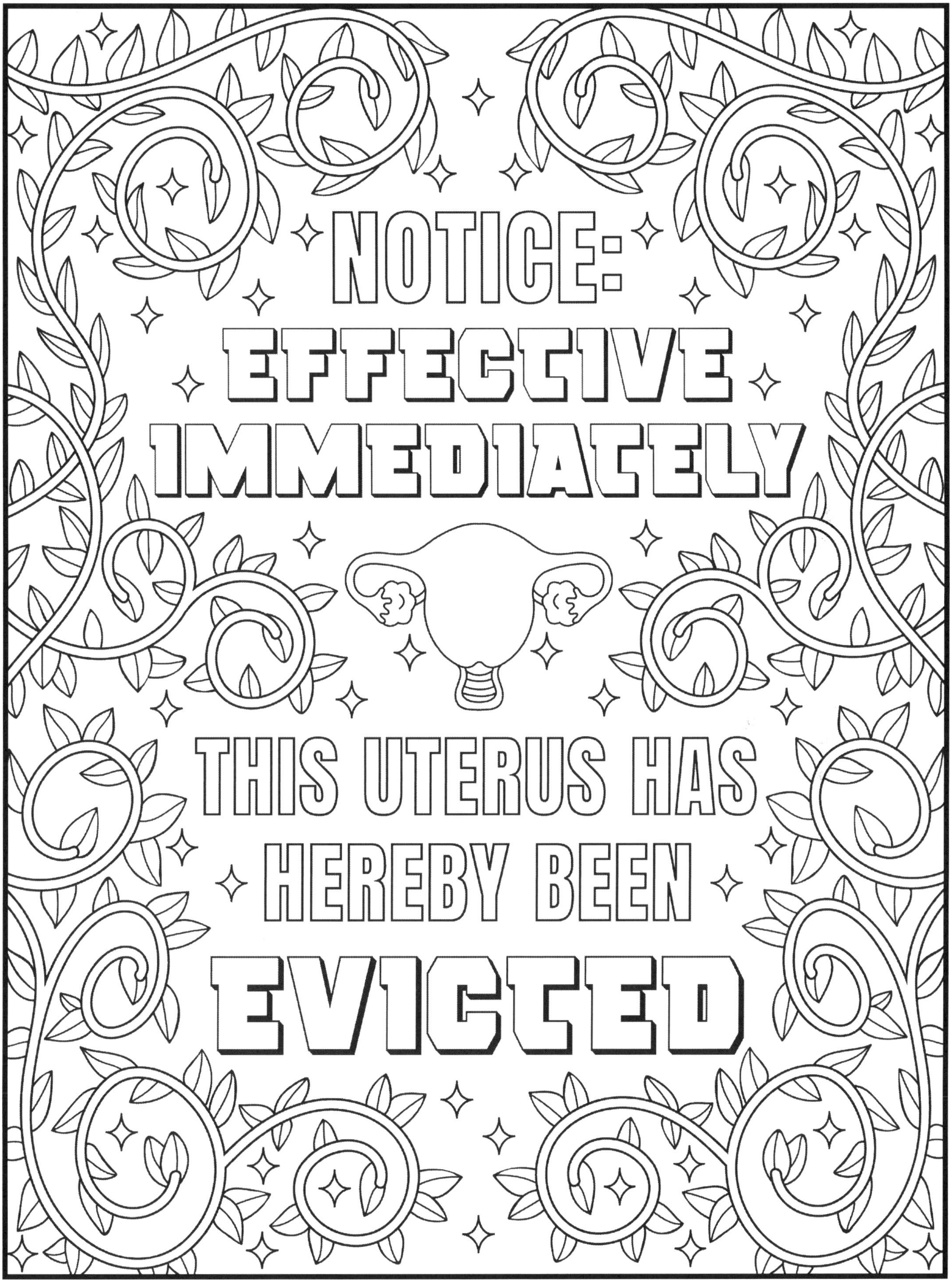
NOTICE:
EFFECTIVE
IMMEDIATELY
THIS UTERUS HAS
HEREBY BEEN
EVICTED

HAVING A

HYSTERECTOMY

Is easy...it's like

RIDING A BIKE

Except the bike is on fire

You're on fire

Everything is on fire

SUDOKU PUZZLES

#1

8	6					3		
4		2			7		8	
	1						7	
		3			9			
2		6				9		
	7							8
5	9			8			2	3
			4	9				7
				6	5	4		1

#2

					1	2		
		8	4				1	
	1	5					9	6
		2			5	9	4	
	8							2
1		9			3			
		3		5			6	4
	5	6		9				
	4						2	9

#3

	1		4	7		2	9	
	2							4
		8		2	9	1	5	
	7		1		8			
	5				2	8	7	
	9		7					
5	3					4		
4	6			8	7			
	8	1	5					6

#4

				8		9	7	
2		5		7			3	
	7		6	3	2		5	4
		4	9					7
9					8	2		5
						3	4	
			5	2	1			
4		1	8					6
					4	5		

#5

				7		5		
	9	2			5		3	
5		7		4			1	2
	8		7	2				
	1				3	9		4
			1					
						3		
9	4		6			2		
	2		4	3		1	6	9

#6

			7	5	3	1		
6		5				7		9
1	7							3
				2	4			
3			9	7		6		
9	2	1						
7				6			4	
	4		5			3	1	7
	1							

#7

		4	7		8			
5			4				7	3
7	2		1	3				
	6				7	4		
	7			5	6		8	
			8	9			2	
		5				6	4	
2	9	7					5	8
		6		7	1		9	2

#8

6			5	8		3		
9						8	1	4
		4	3			7		9
					9		8	
		6	4				2	
	5			9				8
	6	9	8	7			5	1
	3			2				

#9

						2		9
		7	9				4	5
5			7			3	1	
1		5			2	7		
	4		8					
	7				1			
		8	5	9			2	
4							9	6
9			6					7

#10

		2			4	9		6
				6		8	7	
			2				4	
6		4	1					3
					7	4		9
		7	3		6			8
					9	2	8	
7				3		6	9	
				2	1			

#11

				8				9
3	4	7		1				
5					4			
6			5	2				
		8				7		
	1	5						6
4			8			3		
		3	7	5	1	6		4
9			4		6	8		7

#12

	6	7			9			
4		1		5	6		8	
					7			1
	2			3	5			6
				1		9		7
		4						
		5	2		3		6	
		2					7	9
				9		4		

#13

3		2					8	
			4	1	8	3		
	9		3			5	4	
7				8		6	3	2
4					6			
							1	
	8	6						
	7	4	8		3	2	6	
9	3	1			7	4		

#14

1	8	2				7	3	
	6		2			4		
							2	
			7	5		3		9
9		7	8					
3						1		8
2	9						4	
6			3	9				
	7	8	4					

#15

			6	9			1	
			5	4		6		8
	2			3	7		4	
6	1							
2			8		3		5	
3		9	7	5		4	6	
	6						8	
	7			8	4		9	6
4	3		9	1		7		5

#16

				8				1
	6				7	8	2	
		8				7		
	7	1				3		
	8			3	4			2
		6	8		2	5		
	3		4				5	
6						9	1	
			2	5				

#17

	6	9		4		1		
	3					6		9
8					6			
1				9	7		8	5
		4					6	
				1			9	
	9	5	4				1	2
3	1		7		2			
				8	9			

#18

				3	9			8
3		5				9		
					7		3	
1						4		9
4							8	
9		3			1		5	6
	1	2	7	9				3
5		7			4			
	9		2				6	

#19

				9		8		
			2	6		9		
	9	8						4
	4		5					
	5		1			6		
1		7				5		
4		2			7	1		5
7	8		6	1			3	
3				4	2		6	9

#20

1	7				3			5
			6	2			4	
	6							
2			5			9	8	
			7			4		
9	1						6	
			9				1	
7	5				6			
	9	1	4			2	3	

#21

2		8		6				
	7	1	2		9	5		
9	5				7	8	6	
7					2			9
						3	1	
								7
4							2	
8	6	7	1	2		9		5
1					8		7	6

#22

9					7		8	
6					5	7		
8			6		2			
							5	
		9	2					
	7		8	6		2		4
	6			9		1		
3	5		7	2				
4		8			6	3		2

#23

		9	8		6			7
	1							8
	7					9		
				3	8		9	6
6		7		5				1
							8	
7	6	8		2			5	
5		3						2
9		1	4					

#24

		7		2				
6	3					8		
			4					
7		8		1		6		
9	5			8			3	
	6	3		9				
			1		7	5	6	2
				3			7	1
		1	9					3

#25

9			2				3	
			5		6			
6	1	5		3				
		4			9	3		7
3			6		5	8		2
		1		2		9	5	
		7		5	2			
			9	7	4	1		
	3						9	5

#26

9					7			
	3					8		5
4					9			6
7	4				6	9		
6	5	9					4	
		8			5		2	
8		4	9		2	5		
			7	6			8	
			5	8	3	2		4

#27

2			1					
4						9		3
	3				9	1	8	
9				5			7	6
8	6	4			2	5		
	2			9	7	8	6	
	4		2			3		
	7				4			

#28

	2					4	1	
8	4	5						7
		3			7		8	6
		9	1		2			
2			3					1
				7	8			
	5			9		6		4
		8			4		5	
		4		5			7	9

#29

2	6							
	8				9	1		
3	1			5			6	7
6		3				8		
				6			7	9
		2						6
			7	1			2	
	5		2			6	1	
				8	3		9	

#30

1		7		5				4
				9				1
	3			7	2	5		
3	8	4	7					2
	2				4	9		
	7		5	2				
			9				4	
2	4	3	8		6			

#31

		8	3	2				
2	7				5		4	
	3	9				8		
					2		9	4
				9				1
1				6			3	
	1		7					6
					8		7	2
8	5	7				3		

#32

		2	8		9			
					7			
	9	6	3			5		
	3		9					2
9							8	1
7		8					5	
2	4		6		3			
8			7	2	4			
		7			8		1	

#33

								4
	2	4		9		8		1
8	1	6		2	5			
			1			3	2	
		3						9
					2			
				1	6	9	3	2
9			7				1	
	8			4				

#34

9	2		6		1	5		
4			9		5	1		8
	5	3					7	
	4		1	8	3	9		
			7					2
2							5	1
		9		1	6	7		
	3			7	2			

#35

		9		2				
	4		9			6	2	8
					1			
9	5		8					
3	2						4	
		4		5				3
6				4			8	
				8	5		1	6
			7	9		5		

#36

2					6	7		
	1			4			6	
		9	5				2	
			1			8		
4				8			1	5
		6	2	7		3		
	4					5	3	
		5				1		
8							9	2

#37

6			7	8		4	2	
				2	9		6	
	8			4		9		1
	7			1			3	
						5		
	9		8		7		1	
5		8	1	7				
	3				4	2		5
			3					

#38

		2	8		3	6		
7		1		9			8	4
			2					
1		8		5			2	
9			1					
5						8		7
				8			4	6
2		9	4		1		3	
6				7		1		

#39

7	2		4					3
	8	9		5			2	
						7		
2							9	5
			9	4		2		6
	9	7	1				3	
3					6	5		
	7			1	8			
		5					1	

#40

			7		6	5		
5				9				6
6	7			3				9
			9		5			
	8	4		6		2		
				7				
4			6	2			3	
		3	8		7		2	4
	1			4				

Solutions

#1

8	6	7	1	5	2	3	4	9
4	5	2	9	3	7	1	8	6
3	1	9	8	4	6	5	7	2
1	8	3	5	2	9	7	6	4
2	4	6	3	7	8	9	1	5
9	7	5	6	1	4	2	3	8
5	9	4	7	8	1	6	2	3
6	2	1	4	9	3	8	5	7
7	3	8	2	6	5	4	9	1

#2

4	9	7	5	6	1	2	8	3
6	2	8	4	3	9	7	1	5
3	1	5	7	2	8	4	9	6
7	3	2	6	8	5	9	4	1
5	8	4	9	1	7	6	3	2
1	6	9	2	4	3	8	5	7
9	7	3	8	5	2	1	6	4
2	5	6	1	9	4	3	7	8
8	4	1	3	7	6	5	2	9

#3

3	1	5	4	7	6	2	9	8
7	2	9	8	1	5	3	6	4
6	4	8	3	2	9	1	5	7
2	7	6	1	3	8	9	4	5
1	5	4	6	9	2	8	7	3
8	9	3	7	5	4	6	1	2
5	3	7	2	6	1	4	8	9
4	6	2	9	8	7	5	3	1
9	8	1	5	4	3	7	2	6

#4

6	4	3	1	8	5	9	7	2
2	8	5	4	7	9	6	3	1
1	7	9	6	3	2	8	5	4
3	2	4	9	5	6	1	8	7
9	1	7	3	4	8	2	6	5
5	6	8	2	1	7	3	4	9
7	3	6	5	2	1	4	9	8
4	5	1	8	9	3	7	2	6
8	9	2	7	6	4	5	1	3

#5

4	3	8	2	7	1	5	9	6
1	9	2	8	6	5	4	3	7
5	6	7	3	4	9	8	1	2
3	8	9	7	2	4	6	5	1
7	1	6	5	8	3	9	2	4
2	5	4	1	9	6	7	8	3
6	7	1	9	5	2	3	4	8
9	4	3	6	1	8	2	7	5
8	2	5	4	3	7	1	6	9

#6

4	8	9	7	5	3	1	6	2
6	3	5	4	1	2	7	8	9
1	7	2	8	9	6	4	5	3
8	6	7	1	2	4	9	3	5
3	5	4	9	7	8	6	2	1
9	2	1	6	3	5	8	7	4
7	9	3	2	6	1	5	4	8
2	4	6	5	8	9	3	1	7
5	1	8	3	4	7	2	9	6

#7

6	3	4	7	2	8	5	1	9
5	8	1	4	6	9	2	7	3
7	2	9	1	3	5	8	6	4
9	6	8	2	1	7	4	3	5
4	7	2	3	5	6	9	8	1
1	5	3	8	9	4	7	2	6
3	1	5	9	8	2	6	4	7
2	9	7	6	4	3	1	5	8
8	4	6	5	7	1	3	9	2

#8

8	2	3	9	4	1	5	7	6
6	4	1	5	8	7	3	9	2
9	7	5	2	3	6	8	1	4
5	8	4	3	1	2	7	6	9
3	1	2	7	6	9	4	8	5
7	9	6	4	5	8	1	2	3
2	5	7	1	9	4	6	3	8
4	6	9	8	7	3	2	5	1
1	3	8	6	2	5	9	4	7

#9

6	8	4	1	3	5	2	7	9
3	1	7	9	2	8	6	4	5
5	2	9	7	4	6	3	1	8
1	9	5	3	6	2	7	8	4
2	4	6	8	7	9	1	5	3
8	7	3	4	5	1	9	6	2
7	6	8	5	9	3	4	2	1
4	3	1	2	8	7	5	9	6
9	5	2	6	1	4	8	3	7

#10

8	3	2	7	5	4	9	1	6
1	4	5	9	6	3	8	7	2
9	7	6	2	1	8	3	4	5
6	8	4	1	9	2	7	5	3
2	1	3	5	8	7	4	6	9
5	9	7	3	4	6	1	2	8
3	5	1	6	7	9	2	8	4
7	2	8	4	3	5	6	9	1
4	6	9	8	2	1	5	3	7

#11

1	6	2	3	8	5	4	7	9
3	4	7	6	1	9	5	8	2
5	8	9	2	7	4	1	6	3
6	3	4	5	2	7	9	1	8
2	9	8	1	6	3	7	4	5
7	1	5	9	4	8	2	3	6
4	7	6	8	9	2	3	5	1
8	2	3	7	5	1	6	9	4
9	5	1	4	3	6	8	2	7

#12

8	6	7	1	2	9	5	3	4
4	9	1	3	5	6	7	8	2
2	5	3	8	4	7	6	9	1
1	2	9	7	3	5	8	4	6
3	8	6	4	1	2	9	5	7
5	7	4	9	6	8	2	1	3
9	4	5	2	7	3	1	6	8
6	1	2	5	8	4	3	7	9
7	3	8	6	9	1	4	2	5

#13

3	4	2	7	5	9	1	8	6
6	5	7	4	1	8	3	2	9
1	9	8	3	6	2	5	4	7
7	1	5	9	8	4	6	3	2
4	2	3	1	7	6	8	9	5
8	6	9	2	3	5	7	1	4
2	8	6	5	4	1	9	7	3
5	7	4	8	9	3	2	6	1
9	3	1	6	2	7	4	5	8

#14

1	8	2	6	4	9	7	3	5
7	6	5	2	8	3	4	9	1
4	3	9	1	7	5	8	2	6
8	2	4	7	5	1	3	6	9
9	1	7	8	3	6	2	5	4
3	5	6	9	2	4	1	7	8
2	9	3	5	1	8	6	4	7
6	4	1	3	9	7	5	8	2
5	7	8	4	6	2	9	1	3

#15

7	5	4	6	9	8	2	1	3
1	9	3	5	4	2	6	7	8
8	2	6	1	3	7	5	4	9
6	1	5	4	2	9	8	3	7
2	4	7	8	6	3	9	5	1
3	8	9	7	5	1	4	6	2
9	6	2	3	7	5	1	8	4
5	7	1	2	8	4	3	9	6
4	3	8	9	1	6	7	2	5

#16

5	2	7	6	8	3	4	9	1
1	6	3	9	4	7	8	2	5
4	9	8	1	2	5	7	3	6
2	7	1	5	9	6	3	4	8
9	8	5	7	3	4	1	6	2
3	4	6	8	1	2	5	7	9
8	3	9	4	6	1	2	5	7
6	5	2	3	7	8	9	1	4
7	1	4	2	5	9	6	8	3

#17

2	6	9	3	4	5	1	7	8
4	3	7	8	2	1	6	5	9
8	5	1	9	7	6	3	2	4
1	2	3	6	9	7	4	8	5
9	7	4	5	3	8	2	6	1
5	8	6	2	1	4	7	9	3
7	9	5	4	6	3	8	1	2
3	1	8	7	5	2	9	4	6
6	4	2	1	8	9	5	3	7

#18

7	4	1	5	3	9	6	2	8
3	6	5	4	2	8	9	1	7
2	8	9	1	6	7	5	3	4
1	2	8	3	5	6	4	7	9
4	5	6	9	7	2	3	8	1
9	7	3	8	4	1	2	5	6
6	1	2	7	9	5	8	4	3
5	3	7	6	8	4	1	9	2
8	9	4	2	1	3	7	6	5

#19

2	7	1	3	9	4	8	5	6
5	3	4	2	6	8	9	7	1
6	9	8	7	5	1	3	2	4
9	4	6	5	7	3	2	1	8
8	5	3	1	2	9	6	4	7
1	2	7	4	8	6	5	9	3
4	6	2	9	3	7	1	8	5
7	8	9	6	1	5	4	3	2
3	1	5	8	4	2	7	6	9

#20

1	7	9	8	4	3	6	2	5
5	3	8	6	2	7	1	4	9
4	6	2	1	5	9	3	7	8
2	4	7	5	6	1	9	8	3
3	8	6	7	9	2	4	5	1
9	1	5	3	8	4	7	6	2
6	2	4	9	3	8	5	1	7
7	5	3	2	1	6	8	9	4
8	9	1	4	7	5	2	3	6

#21

2	4	8	5	6	3	7	9	1
6	7	1	2	8	9	5	4	3
9	5	3	4	1	7	8	6	2
7	1	4	3	5	2	6	8	9
5	8	2	7	9	6	3	1	4
3	9	6	8	4	1	2	5	7
4	3	9	6	7	5	1	2	8
8	6	7	1	2	4	9	3	5
1	2	5	9	3	8	4	7	6

#22

9	2	5	1	3	7	4	8	6
6	3	4	9	8	5	7	2	1
8	1	7	6	4	2	5	3	9
2	8	6	4	7	1	9	5	3
1	4	9	2	5	3	8	6	7
5	7	3	8	6	9	2	1	4
7	6	2	3	9	8	1	4	5
3	5	1	7	2	4	6	9	8
4	9	8	5	1	6	3	7	2

#23

2	3	9	8	4	6	5	1	7
4	1	5	2	9	7	6	3	8
8	7	6	5	1	3	9	2	4
1	5	4	7	3	8	2	9	6
6	8	7	9	5	2	3	4	1
3	9	2	1	6	4	7	8	5
7	6	8	3	2	1	4	5	9
5	4	3	6	8	9	1	7	2
9	2	1	4	7	5	8	6	3

#24

4	9	7	8	2	1	3	5	6
6	3	2	5	7	9	8	1	4
8	1	5	4	6	3	7	2	9
7	2	8	3	1	4	6	9	5
9	5	4	6	8	2	1	3	7
1	6	3	7	9	5	2	4	8
3	8	9	1	4	7	5	6	2
5	4	6	2	3	8	9	7	1
2	7	1	9	5	6	4	8	3

#25

9	4	8	2	1	7	5	3	6
7	2	3	5	9	6	4	8	1
6	1	5	4	3	8	2	7	9
2	5	4	1	8	9	3	6	7
3	7	9	6	4	5	8	1	2
8	6	1	7	2	3	9	5	4
1	9	7	3	5	2	6	4	8
5	8	6	9	7	4	1	2	3
4	3	2	8	6	1	7	9	5

#26

9	6	1	8	5	7	4	3	2
2	3	7	6	4	1	8	9	5
4	8	5	3	2	9	7	1	6
7	4	2	1	3	6	9	5	8
6	5	9	2	7	8	3	4	1
3	1	8	4	9	5	6	2	7
8	7	4	9	1	2	5	6	3
5	2	3	7	6	4	1	8	9
1	9	6	5	8	3	2	7	4

#27

1	8	6	9	4	3	7	2	5
2	9	3	1	7	5	6	4	8
4	5	7	8	2	6	9	1	3
7	3	5	4	6	9	1	8	2
9	1	2	3	5	8	4	7	6
8	6	4	7	1	2	5	3	9
3	2	1	5	9	7	8	6	4
6	4	9	2	8	1	3	5	7
5	7	8	6	3	4	2	9	1

#28

6	2	7	5	8	9	4	1	3
8	4	5	6	1	3	9	2	7
1	9	3	4	2	7	5	8	6
5	7	9	1	6	2	3	4	8
2	8	6	3	4	5	7	9	1
4	3	1	9	7	8	2	6	5
7	5	2	8	9	1	6	3	4
9	6	8	7	3	4	1	5	2
3	1	4	2	5	6	8	7	9

#29

2	6	7	4	3	1	9	8	5
4	8	5	6	7	9	1	3	2
3	1	9	8	5	2	4	6	7
6	7	3	9	2	5	8	4	1
5	4	1	3	6	8	2	7	9
8	9	2	1	4	7	3	5	6
9	3	4	7	1	6	5	2	8
7	5	8	2	9	4	6	1	3
1	2	6	5	8	3	7	9	4

#30

1	9	7	6	5	8	3	2	4
8	5	2	4	9	3	6	7	1
4	3	6	1	7	2	5	8	9
3	8	4	7	6	9	1	5	2
5	2	1	3	8	4	9	6	7
6	7	9	5	2	1	4	3	8
9	6	5	2	4	7	8	1	3
7	1	8	9	3	5	2	4	6
2	4	3	8	1	6	7	9	5

#31

5	4	8	3	2	9	1	6	7
2	7	1	6	8	5	9	4	3
6	3	9	4	7	1	8	2	5
7	8	5	1	3	2	6	9	4
3	2	6	8	9	4	7	5	1
1	9	4	5	6	7	2	3	8
9	1	2	7	5	3	4	8	6
4	6	3	9	1	8	5	7	2
8	5	7	2	4	6	3	1	9

#32

4	7	2	8	5	9	1	6	3
5	8	3	1	6	7	4	2	9
1	9	6	3	4	2	5	7	8
6	3	1	9	8	5	7	4	2
9	5	4	2	7	6	3	8	1
7	2	8	4	3	1	9	5	6
2	4	5	6	1	3	8	9	7
8	1	9	7	2	4	6	3	5
3	6	7	5	9	8	2	1	4

#33

7	3	9	6	8	1	2	5	4
5	2	4	3	9	7	8	6	1
8	1	6	4	2	5	7	9	3
6	9	8	1	7	4	3	2	5
2	7	3	5	6	8	1	4	9
1	4	5	9	3	2	6	8	7
4	5	7	8	1	6	9	3	2
9	6	2	7	5	3	4	1	8
3	8	1	2	4	9	5	7	6

#34

3	1	5	8	4	7	2	9	6
9	2	8	6	3	1	5	4	7
4	6	7	9	2	5	1	3	8
1	5	3	2	6	9	8	7	4
7	4	2	1	8	3	9	6	5
8	9	6	7	5	4	3	1	2
2	7	4	3	9	8	6	5	1
5	8	9	4	1	6	7	2	3
6	3	1	5	7	2	4	8	9

#35

7	6	9	4	2	8	3	5	1
5	4	1	9	7	3	6	2	8
2	8	3	5	6	1	4	9	7
9	5	6	8	3	4	1	7	2
3	2	8	6	1	7	9	4	5
1	7	4	2	5	9	8	6	3
6	3	5	1	4	2	7	8	9
4	9	7	3	8	5	2	1	6
8	1	2	7	9	6	5	3	4

#36

2	3	4	9	1	6	7	5	8
5	1	8	7	4	2	9	6	3
7	6	9	5	3	8	4	2	1
3	5	2	1	9	4	8	7	6
4	9	7	6	8	3	2	1	5
1	8	6	2	7	5	3	4	9
6	4	1	8	2	9	5	3	7
9	2	5	3	6	7	1	8	4
8	7	3	4	5	1	6	9	2

#37

6	5	9	7	8	1	4	2	3
3	4	1	5	2	9	7	6	8
7	8	2	6	4	3	9	5	1
2	7	6	4	1	5	8	3	9
8	1	3	2	9	6	5	4	7
4	9	5	8	3	7	6	1	2
5	6	8	1	7	2	3	9	4
1	3	7	9	6	4	2	8	5
9	2	4	3	5	8	1	7	6

#38

4	5	2	8	1	3	6	7	9
7	3	1	5	9	6	2	8	4
8	9	6	2	4	7	3	5	1
1	6	8	7	5	4	9	2	3
9	2	7	1	3	8	4	6	5
5	4	3	6	2	9	8	1	7
3	1	5	9	8	2	7	4	6
2	7	9	4	6	1	5	3	8
6	8	4	3	7	5	1	9	2

#39

7	2	1	4	8	9	6	5	3
6	8	9	3	5	7	4	2	1
4	5	3	6	2	1	7	8	9
2	4	6	8	7	3	1	9	5
1	3	8	9	4	5	2	7	6
5	9	7	1	6	2	8	3	4
3	1	2	7	9	6	5	4	8
9	7	4	5	1	8	3	6	2
8	6	5	2	3	4	9	1	7

#40

3	4	9	7	1	6	5	8	2
5	2	1	4	9	8	3	7	6
6	7	8	5	3	2	4	1	9
2	3	6	9	8	5	7	4	1
7	8	4	1	6	3	2	9	5
1	9	5	2	7	4	8	6	3
4	5	7	6	2	1	9	3	8
9	6	3	8	5	7	1	2	4
8	1	2	3	4	9	6	5	7

WORD SEARCH

H	J	L	N	Z	B	P	F	D	Y	T	P	P	E	N	I	T	E	N	T	Y	Y	J
J	S	V	J	Z	C	O	R	R	E	C	T	Z	A	G	V	R	V	S	T	W	D	Z
H	Y	S	T	E	R	E	C	T	O	M	Y	H	K	Q	W	K	Y	J	U	W	L	A
O	I	L	P	N	M	O	T	D	P	J	A	N	O	Y	Q	X	C	K	E	N	I	G
Q	O	C	S	L	C	N	U	T	J	K	S	C	E	R	V	I	X	Z	F	X	Y	I
B	J	Q	H	S	O	P	H	I	S	T	I	C	A	T	E	D	K	W	B	X	F	H
T	O	Z	P	L	Z	F	C	C	D	L	N	X	B	V	G	L	T	R	Y	A	P	E
P	W	H	B	H	W	M	X	K	B	X	G	X	Y	C	Y	V	H	L	R	I	B	A
Y	P	A	M	I	O	S	M	G	X	G	L	Y	Z	Z	Z	D	H	S	A	O	C	K
H	B	W	C	H	M	F	N	X	R	A	C	I	A	L	T	O	P	A	S	K	C	C
L	J	N	W	O	B	K	M	L	J	J	Y	V	I	Z	U	M	V	D	P	K	U	W
F	C	G	Y	K	X	P	E	T	J	H	S	U	C	F	R	I	E	M	Y	S	R	X
Q	A	B	O	R	I	G	I	N	A	L	U	T	I	L	G	N	W	I	Y	T	E	K
R	D	E	T	H	E	R	E	A	L	M	J	E	K	T	O	E	S	T	O	R	H	W
O	E	N	P	L	P	C	E	F	D	D	C	R	T	T	V	E	Y	C	X	C	C	Y
M	A	V	V	H	O	S	P	I	T	A	L	U	Y	A	A	R	V	X	R	Y	V	Z
P	D	M	M	Q	U	W	J	G	Q	N	W	S	J	M	R	I	S	N	A	I	L	T
S	M	D	K	W	M	M	H	O	J	J	P	C	J	T	Y	N	A	U	Z	O	F	T
D	N	W	U	B	O	B	E	D	S	L	B	L	X	O	C	G	T	Q	D	V	A	T
W	Y	Y	S	S	S	Z	K	L	P	T	I	N	S	U	R	A	N	C	E	F	P	F
U	V	E	Y	O	U	C	U	Y	A	D	V	M	E	W	V	V	H	T	K	E	H	X
W	F	X	G	W	Q	H	T	C	C	O	K	Z	J	B	A	W	D	Y	Q	O	C	R
P	F	G	R	B	B	I	K	N	E	S	F	Z	N	A	I	R	G	W	S	A	X	X

DOMINEERING, RACIAL, SOPHISTICATED, UTERUS, CERVIX, BAWDY, ETHEREAL, OVARY, SNAIL, ADMIT, PENITENT, HYSTERECTOMY, CORRECT, RASPY, GODLY, SPACE, AIR, HOSPITAL, ABORIGINAL, DEAD, INSURANCE, WOMB, CURE

W	O	W	E	G	R	H	A	P	P	Y	H	K	D	G	G	H	K	W	H	B	K	B
R	F	T	V	N	N	W	P	S	Y	C	B	X	A	I	F	F	L	K	S	P	V	U
E	U	E	X	B	M	Q	R	P	V	G	D	P	S	P	O	O	K	Y	P	H	B	S
L	B	I	O	C	K	E	E	A	X	M	O	Y	J	R	Y	D	N	X	F	S	A	Y
A	Q	I	Z	B	E	D	G	Q	U	J	R	E	P	L	Y	U	D	G	Z	D	S	G
T	M	H	Z	J	S	Y	N	D	W	T	L	A	H	A	F	Q	O	E	E	D	K	H
I	F	S	V	S	E	R	A	E	V	C	U	X	U	E	N	C	H	A	N	T	E	D
O	C	E	L	N	D	P	N	A	U	R	E	T	H	R	A	X	O	H	Q	N	T	V
N	V	M	L	C	B	S	C	L	W	F	E	T	C	H	C	Z	D	O	Q	L	B	Y
W	G	P	H	I	T	G	Y	Q	J	G	S	G	S	R	B	A	V	U	J	A	A	Z
H	C	K	Z	A	A	Y	V	H	A	L	L	O	W	E	D	T	T	S	Y	E	L	X
I	M	A	G	I	N	A	R	Y	J	K	J	U	O	W	C	T	X	E	W	W	L	O
Y	B	K	N	B	G	F	X	N	D	E	Q	U	W	D	P	E	L	K	H	T	A	V
C	N	T	Y	U	Y	E	J	I	N	B	O	O	R	P	U	N	Q	F	Q	K	D	S
F	E	R	T	I	L	I	Z	A	T	I	O	N	H	I	L	D	M	H	N	K	U	M
W	Z	F	Y	S	W	L	C	Q	A	S	L	Q	J	H	P	N	R	A	I	S	E	N
R	L	K	X	N	U	H	H	N	N	X	D	Z	F	P	P	Z	G	F	X	S	F	S
D	D	A	S	W	E	A	T	E	R	B	S	E	P	T	X	J	E	U	Q	W	N	Z
J	S	U	R	G	E	R	Y	E	Z	F	C	C	D	E	V	G	H	Y	G	T	U	V
B	O	T	P	N	B	S	X	W	F	E	A	F	L	N	Y	T	F	V	Q	I	A	M
B	I	P	I	M	I	G	H	T	Y	R	R	P	U	A	P	O	I	K	G	W	G	V
I	H	S	E	G	A	T	G	D	P	K	E	L	J	S	P	Q	I	O	H	U	D	U
K	B	M	E	N	S	U	R	A	T	I	O	N	P	Q	E	C	Z	R	N	D	H	C

REPLY, SURGERY, URETHRA, RAISE, MIGHTY, ENCHANTED, IMAGINARY, ATTEND, SWEATER, MENSURATION, TAN, FERTILIZATION, FETCH, HOUSE, SPOOKY, HAPPY, PREGNANCY, HALLOWED, BASKETBALL, RELATION, SCARE, BUSY, TANGY

T	H	H	F	E	T	U	S	D	J	O	H	N	W	K	U	P	A	P	J	O	I	X
S	C	Y	M	N	B	O	A	S	T	M	N	L	H	P	U	E	N	V	I	S	Z	I
G	U	T	J	R	H	Q	E	N	G	W	A	N	T	S	X	L	Y	S	I	F	V	I
M	F	P	Y	U	P	M	A	B	M	B	X	U	B	L	W	V	J	F	M	T	S	E
M	I	O	B	P	V	A	C	C	I	N	E	Q	R	E	F	I	P	T	T	Y	R	X
D	Y	S	F	U	N	C	T	I	O	N	A	L	I	Y	S	S	T	U	M	P	P	J
G	C	G	H	U	P	N	V	Y	A	H	C	B	E	I	R	G	R	A	P	E	S	L
H	W	U	E	W	J	K	I	Y	G	H	N	O	F	A	Q	C	U	W	M	W	V	E
Y	V	H	I	M	T	M	X	M	N	V	M	M	A	T	C	H	W	O	R	X	N	T
I	U	V	Z	Z	D	I	Y	D	I	S	A	P	P	E	A	R	D	G	A	E	L	T
D	A	R	N	Z	L	M	H	V	N	L	D	E	L	D	P	T	W	X	J	R	V	E
U	O	A	S	D	M	R	O	P	R	Z	L	Q	X	N	M	D	M	W	Z	I	T	R
J	J	V	K	Z	P	X	Y	A	X	A	U	U	N	K	E	M	P	T	G	P	E	B
E	I	I	F	A	R	O	D	G	E	G	I	U	O	R	A	H	O	P	F	E	U	B
U	Z	H	H	G	I	J	L	C	T	R	I	T	A	U	G	Y	K	O	J	E	T	J
S	K	C	M	E	V	U	S	L	Y	E	F	E	Z	B	S	D	V	P	I	Z	L	I
J	U	J	A	G	A	X	X	A	F	E	R	L	Z	R	N	O	E	M	B	R	Y	O
K	J	U	F	G	T	Q	E	M	V	M	N	O	L	L	D	L	N	M	P	B	G	Q
J	O	R	E	S	E	N	O	N	D	E	S	C	R	I	P	T	O	B	C	X	A	S
Y	U	R	M	C	Q	T	P	O	L	N	B	K	H	Q	C	E	M	Y	S	A	X	J
G	G	Y	A	U	W	Y	K	K	X	T	P	I	H	K	S	Q	O	F	L	N	W	R
V	Q	C	L	O	A	B	S	M	O	G	G	Y	X	V	E	M	U	K	O	A	U	V
C	V	D	E	B	W	I	J	L	S	S	S	X	X	T	P	L	S	S	X	V	Q	H

MATCH, VENOMOUS, NONDESCRIPT, BOAST, CLAM, DYSFUNCTIONAL, ANTS, RUB, EGGS, BRIEF, UNKEMPT, AGREEMENT, FEMALE, SMOGGY, PRIVATE, VACCINE, GRAPE, LETTER, EMBRYO, RIPE, FETUS, DISAPPEAR, PELVIS

S	T	R	A	P	G	V	X	D	Y	C	Y	O	P	E	U	E	G	O	R	G
F	A	K	H	J	K	E	F	Q	P	M	U	K	V	C	W	U	U	E	G	D
W	Y	N	W	P	J	M	D	Y	P	H	C	Y	Q	R	H	P	A	H	L	T
Q	B	U	K	D	M	N	L	V	C	E	I	S	W	F	W	B	R	W	R	H
R	Y	Z	O	X	T	R	I	M	M	O	T	H	E	R	X	S	A	S	R	H
V	I	P	X	M	Y	G	Z	L	N	A	M	E	V	B	A	E	N	K	E	K
E	I	A	C	J	W	A	V	E	F	L	C	J	L	U	K	I	T	S	C	K
E	S	R	Y	U	O	D	U	Q	I	O	K	K	I	R	C	B	E	R	B	P
W	G	T	N	W	L	H	L	J	G	Y	R	Q	T	Y	F	R	E	R	P	C
F	I	N	A	Y	F	R	A	N	T	I	C	W	T	U	E	O	M	I	X	J
E	L	E	V	P	X	P	S	I	Q	C	O	L	L	A	R	B	Z	Q	F	P
Q	E	R	E	B	U	G	U	S	T	Y	H	O	E	A	Z	G	N	L	L	F
L	A	O	B	J	E	C	T	S	A	A	K	J	E	W	R	J	E	X	F	R
K	T	T	R	I	T	G	J	J	N	P	E	A	C	E	F	U	L	F	R	E
O	H	J	A	B	R	X	C	F	C	H	Z	J	B	F	W	S	L	E	E	Y
H	E	S	I	N	A	R	S	N	W	B	Z	T	B	Y	V	O	L	H	Q	M
A	R	S	N	I	D	J	W	X	V	U	B	R	Q	K	K	Z	Z	A	U	K
V	Z	B	Y	J	R	J	I	U	I	N	T	E	R	F	E	R	E	R	E	O
R	E	S	T	O	O	N	N	Q	X	Y	E	A	S	X	I	R	F	S	N	V
K	J	P	T	J	P	V	G	U	X	K	V	T	Q	X	F	J	I	H	T	D
H	F	T	S	N	I	N	T	E	R	E	S	T	I	N	G	T	S	F	B	L

COLLAR, SWING, MOTHER, INTERESTING, DROP, FREQUENT, STRAP, GUARANTEE, NAME, TREAT, OBJECT, BRAINY, HARSH, REST, WAVE, GUSTY, PEACEFUL, FRANTIC, LITTLE, PARTNER, LEATHER, INTERFERE, BURY

P	Z	R	L	Y	G	D	W	H	Y	O	Q	F	G	H	D	W	C
H	Z	B	R	L	Q	G	C	S	C	A	Z	F	A	I	R	A	S
Y	V	I	S	O	H	D	Z	W	O	D	V	E	T	N	U	N	V
S	O	F	P	P	E	K	Y	K	R	R	R	G	T	P	D	I	J
I	L	O	O	S	D	H	F	G	N	S	T	R	A	N	G	E	X
C	C	I	T	I	U	E	M	H	S	E	Z	U	C	Z	W	W	M
A	A	A	T	D	C	A	C	Y	W	U	G	R	H	M	W	M	C
L	N	P	E	E	A	V	W	R	A	P	A	Y	M	P	W	S	R
I	O	S	D	D	T	Y	A	M	A	Z	I	N	G	U	Q	I	Z
Z	Z	V	I	O	E	W	K	H	L	O	N	G	I	N	G	S	Z
M	E	K	L	U	D	Z	D	A	R	F	O	O	L	G	B	S	T
F	R	O	G	S	F	D	F	N	N	Q	M	T	X	N	D	U	C
L	A	V	I	S	H	Z	X	D	W	N	E	L	R	P	O	P	F
S	L	E	R	E	C	T	L	S	N	A	M	P	W	E	C	P	W
B	M	L	E	C	S	M	R	O	O	Q	O	O	M	T	T	O	N
A	V	B	V	F	F	P	P	M	E	Q	R	U	L	S	O	S	E
Q	D	Y	H	B	F	G	V	E	D	I	Y	R	J	Y	R	E	N
T	P	U	L	E	E	K	Z	P	Q	P	O	E	Y	Z	S	R	H

LAVISH, FOOL, CORN, SPOTTED, HEAVY, WRAP, POUR, HANDSOME, ERECT, AMAZING, LONGING, LOPSIDED, STRANGE, ATTACH, SUPPOSE, DOCTORS, MEMORY, PHYSICAL, FAIR, EDUCATED, VOLCANO, PETS, FROGS

Q	N	F	A	I	T	H	F	U	L	J	I	I	S	H	C	H	K	Z	H
H	L	T	J	Z	A	T	D	R	Y	K	Z	E	F	J	H	F	E	T	H
I	L	S	A	G	T	E	F	F	I	C	I	E	N	T	I	R	T	R	L
B	L	U	S	H	M	V	Q	Z	S	C	Q	Q	R	O	E	D	A	V	R
O	Z	F	U	F	D	Y	U	S	J	B	E	K	Y	L	F	B	A	B	Y
D	Y	G	N	R	U	F	J	O	C	Z	S	G	F	U	I	T	R	E	Z
D	S	S	U	Y	G	S	H	O	E	E	D	I	Q	S	U	H	Q	Z	W
Y	X	H	M	Q	W	O	G	U	B	X	U	C	X	F	E	U	B	Z	L
Q	U	A	R	T	E	R	R	A	F	Z	Y	Q	S	O	R	N	R	Z	T
J	W	R	O	N	G	M	A	A	G	B	I	U	T	Z	M	D	E	T	V
K	C	L	U	O	J	O	N	J	T	B	G	E	R	T	K	E	S	C	G
B	W	O	N	E	W	T	D	E	S	O	O	E	E	W	V	R	C	Y	T
V	E	Z	H	P	U	I	I	F	C	R	V	N	T	L	N	I	U	V	S
X	L	M	A	R	B	O	O	L	V	R	E	N	C	Z	F	N	E	E	C
G	L	T	R	A	E	N	S	K	L	O	R	Y	H	C	L	G	I	K	I
R	-	L	M	Z	L	L	E	L	U	W	N	T	S	T	E	W	X	L	S
Q	O	A	Z	Z	A	E	N	M	V	D	O	R	E	V	Q	M	J	W	S
B	F	Y	C	Y	G	S	J	R	H	W	R	L	H	G	T	W	P	V	O
Z	F	T	P	V	G	S	B	F	R	R	A	D	I	A	T	E	W	C	R
W	F	E	I	I	M	J	H	J	T	U	Y	H	L	Z	A	G	E	Q	S

FAITHFUL, SHOE, QUEEN, THUNDERING, CHIEF, GOVERNOR, QUARTER, MOTIONLESS, SCISSORS, EFFICIENT, BABY, ONE, WRONG, BLUSH, GRANDIOSE, WELL-OFF, DRY, ODD, STRETCH, STEW, BORROW, RESCUE, RADIATE

U	D	E	B	W	Z	T	I	X	F	P	M	K	L	B	Y	U	G	X	T	C
D	U	S	T	Y	P	I	O	B	A	B	Q	F	F	A	S	S	C	J	J	S
W	H	S	O	O	Q	C	H	C	J	Y	B	L	P	Q	K	P	D	M	V	J
M	O	N	D	V	P	K	S	J	Y	Y	Y	K	F	I	W	Q	J	S	C	P
I	U	P	R	I	V	E	R	Q	G	J	F	F	K	M	E	Z	K	S	T	Y
D	S	J	F	P	I	T	K	P	X	Z	C	J	E	O	X	E	L	Y	T	V
J	F	S	T	U	P	I	D	C	T	R	U	L	E	L	P	C	P	F	O	J
F	P	B	B	O	T	Y	A	F	T	E	R	M	A	T	H	T	P	T	V	O
J	T	A	O	D	H	V	T	E	F	F	I	C	A	C	I	O	U	S	M	Y
R	O	T	T	S	R	Y	G	G	S	L	Z	P	W	W	T	R	N	L	C	O
X	U	H	T	L	O	O	K	A	J	E	U	Z	G	R	P	L	C	M	M	U
N	C	E	L	H	A	K	R	R	P	C	Y	C	M	B	O	R	H	C	S	S
M	H	N	E	T	T	W	A	Y	A	T	C	M	Z	V	T	A	P	Y	L	S
X	V	J	B	Q	J	Z	V	A	S	I	N	J	U	R	E	E	E	F	E	J
I	E	K	Z	S	F	J	T	Q	S	G	V	J	M	M	N	U	R	E	E	O
C	H	E	M	I	C	A	L	T	E	U	W	P	U	D	O	M	F	J	T	Z
R	E	L	X	M	B	X	I	G	N	E	G	I	G	W	Y	L	E	O	Y	G
B	M	Z	Z	W	O	L	C	K	G	I	G	Y	Q	D	W	H	C	M	F	X
R	J	G	I	O	X	H	K	L	E	Z	F	N	N	H	M	J	T	L	T	G
E	Y	W	Q	E	V	W	V	V	R	S	B	Y	L	B	A	L	A	N	C	E
M	G	O	Q	R	Q	U	U	T	P	Q	T	C	U	T	D	L	A	U	A	H

SLEET, TOUCH, POT, CHEMICAL, JOYOUS, BALANCE, STUPID, TICKET, REFLECT, EFFICACIOUS, PERFECT, BATHE, AFTERMATH, THROAT, PASSENGER, INJURE, BOTTLE, LOOK, RIVER, MUG, CUT, WAY, DUSTY

Z	V	G	M	L	B	P	Z	W	T	F	I	T	P	J	D	W	Y	N	U
Q	P	Q	G	V	S	I	A	I	S	Z	M	P	R	O	F	I	T	G	Z
M	W	K	I	Q	M	P	G	N	R	W	P	W	F	L	O	W	E	R	Y
N	Q	S	Y	J	W	E	P	D	Z	X	R	B	A	E	L	I	T	E	H
O	B	T	S	N	T	U	X	O	G	S	E	R	E	K	B	O	I	X	Y
V	D	N	G	D	C	J	C	W	K	K	S	W	U	S	K	I	N	D	T
H	A	D	S	T	U	B	L	O	O	D	S	X	W	V	G	P	B	H	J
Q	R	C	C	G	J	I	T	T	E	R	Y	X	Y	G	U	N	C	E	L
S	U	U	R	L	C	O	M	M	I	T	T	E	E	Q	A	K	N	M	R
Y	T	V	I	S	R	K	C	Y	J	W	M	U	D	Y	V	J	L	B	A
M	A	D	B	X	V	B	U	B	O	R	I	N	G	T	V	U	H	B	P
C	S	V	B	R	W	L	P	W	J	U	G	G	L	E	H	O	U	Z	J
G	T	C	L	I	M	O	H	X	A	F	R	A	I	D	K	S	C	N	H
A	E	I	E	A	R	I	T	H	M	E	T	I	C	O	W	S	H	E	U
L	L	P	I	L	R	T	X	P	A	R	C	E	L	V	X	I	I	Q	N
C	E	Z	R	B	Q	I	G	X	M	A	R	K	E	T	R	F	L	W	I
J	S	B	L	U	E	-	E	Y	E	D	G	R	I	Y	K	I	Y	W	T
V	S	O	A	B	Z	K	Y	X	Z	W	D	E	J	F	P	E	V	T	I
W	K	E	P	R	A	C	T	I	C	E	C	T	V	E	W	D	E	O	A
J	E	I	M	Z	W	A	T	C	H	Q	R	C	Q	V	T	Q	B	T	S

PARCEL, JITTERY, BORING, PIPE, JUGGLE, PROFIT, MARKET, OSSIFIED, IMPRESS, SCRIBBLE, BLOOD, FLOWERY, SKIN, ARITHMETIC, COMMITTEE, AFRAID, PRACTICE, BLUE-EYED, TASTELESS, WATCH, WINDOW, UNIT, ELITE

B	H	E	Z	H	I	F	R	V	K	R	M	N	Z	G	V	F	O	H	E	G
J	W	Z	K	I	B	F	L	Y	I	N	G	K	N	M	X	X	S	A	L	S
Z	C	L	O	N	G	-	T	E	R	M	W	A	X	G	I	Q	G	A	O	F
R	X	P	G	O	B	S	E	R	V	A	T	I	O	N	S	U	L	Y	M	I
Q	R	O	Z	T	M	E	I	M	I	N	O	R	N	Z	A	E	Q	A	J	H
Y	E	P	P	R	S	S	H	U	G	G	H	J	X	H	T	T	S	P	T	Z
U	C	E	H	C	W	O	F	Y	T	A	P	P	E	A	R	E	Q	G	H	B
V	O	N	C	S	C	L	E	V	E	L	A	K	S	I	Q	V	B	C	I	L
X	R	A	R	G	U	E	G	U	C	W	X	G	A	F	G	F	P	A	R	E
Z	D	W	S	X	P	D	S	A	N	J	O	M	V	Q	M	F	M	L	S	R
T	N	S	U	I	N	C	Z	K	O	A	L	O	O	D	I	Q	D	C	T	C
R	Q	N	T	A	R	T	N	V	R	R	E	U	R	U	C	B	H	U	Y	P
A	J	J	K	D	U	G	Y	P	T	M	A	N	Y	S	E	R	N	L	T	B
D	X	I	T	L	G	F	R	G	H	G	Z	T	Z	I	Z	U	A	A	W	V
E	A	K	R	P	I	S	A	K	A	M	E	A	K	S	N	H	X	T	L	O
P	P	K	E	J	D	G	Z	K	F	L	U	I	I	T	J	A	V	E	S	B
I	K	F	P	H	D	O	K	F	I	F	S	N	M	E	E	Q	T	O	Q	P
B	C	A	E	A	Y	S	D	M	T	B	G	O	P	R	T	P	F	D	M	L
F	X	S	A	U	R	A	B	B	I	T	S	U	J	S	N	Y	F	T	X	J
V	A	T	T	N	O	H	E	Q	D	J	M	S	H	O	V	H	U	I	W	J
W	Z	Y	N	T	W	Y	Q	K	S	Y	P	A	V	T	U	Z	O	I	J	I

SAVORY, REPEAT, ARGUE, TART, LYING, MINOR, CALCULATE, MOUNTAINOUS, APPEAR, LONG-TERM, THIRSTY, TRADE, SISTERS, HUG, OBSERVATION, RECORD, MICE, HAUNT, FAST, RABBITS, GIDDY, NORTH, LEVEL

X	A	N	V	Y	N	S	Y	R	T	F	D	Y	P	I	C	T	U	R	E	X	V	N
H	L	V	D	I	V	B	U	A	U	K	W	P	O	E	J	D	A	M	B	R	Z	S
N	Q	U	I	Y	L	T	R	I	L	A	R	Q	F	H	W	X	B	F	T	I	S	L
W	S	G	S	D	L	D	B	Z	R	U	D	L	I	Z	F	B	Y	L	G	J	L	L
B	K	A	I	G	E	Y	C	F	K	G	I	N	F	L	E	H	Y	R	E	G	L	D
U	B	V	L	P	E	Y	C	G	A	H	M	L	L	N	Z	Y	G	D	T	V	F	B
O	S	R	L	A	Q	U	A	T	I	C	E	J	M	R	Q	Y	E	U	T	F	S	M
P	Q	T	U	J	S	U	R	P	R	I	S	E	C	A	U	S	N	L	V	I	F	A
P	T	T	S	A	F	V	D	X	C	U	W	P	Y	P	E	N	E	L	C	N	X	U
Y	R	K	I	I	F	S	O	D	P	M	S	R	Z	I	L	G	R	G	S	O	U	L
R	E	H	O	C	Z	E	V	X	A	S	U	F	Q	D	N	P	G	T	T	H	A	S
G	I	G	N	Q	Q	B	E	L	I	M	I	T	F	X	K	F	E	V	R	L	A	M
L	Y	D	E	G	K	U	N	D	R	E	S	S	A	Y	R	H	T	H	A	W	C	E
R	X	B	D	O	H	W	P	H	J	W	X	L	N	U	A	R	I	Z	I	F	T	L
D	A	A	D	A	C	R	I	D	R	S	T	A	B	D	K	L	C	W	G	C	I	L
R	J	Z	F	A	C	P	I	W	L	R	M	U	F	N	R	D	B	K	H	H	V	U
B	F	E	S	Z	Y	I	Z	T	D	T	I	G	A	A	T	V	V	H	T	F	I	N
U	Q	B	B	B	N	C	M	H	M	Z	T	H	B	D	B	J	S	M	E	A	T	W
U	U	D	S	K	I	A	X	Y	P	R	E	A	U	R	U	L	E	B	O	A	Y	E
T	M	L	C	D	C	Y	D	G	E	V	P	B	H	I	L	L	-	F	A	T	E	D
K	V	C	U	A	A	U	C	R	N	S	P	L	J	C	F	P	Y	J	Y	W	N	I
W	T	P	T	S	L	N	Q	G	K	G	M	E	P	Z	L	B	P	O	W	D	E	R
F	H	Y	H	M	Y	E	F	Q	O	C	O	S	I	W	B	U	O	H	E	F	C	J

STRAIGHT, CYNICAL, PEN, DIME, DISILLUSIONED, SURPRISE, ILL-FATED, POWDER, DULL, LIMIT, UNDRESS, LAUGHABLE, ENERGETIC, OVEN, PICTURE, AQUATIC, RULE, ACTIVITY, MEAT, SMELL, PICAYUNE, RAPID, ACRID

Solutions

H J L N Z B P F D Y T P P E N I T E N T Y Y J

J S V J Z C O R R E C T Z A G V R V S T W D Z

H Y S T E R E C T O M Y H K Q W K Y J U W L A

O I L P N M O T D P J A N O Y Q X C K E N I G

Q O C S L C N U T J K S C E R V I X Z F X Y I

B J Q H S O P H I S T I C A T E D K W B X F H

T O Z P L Z F C C D L N X B V G L T R Y A P E

P W H B H W M X K B X G X Y C Y V H L R I B A

Y P A M I O S M G X G L Y Z Z Z D H S A O C K

H B W C H M F N X R A C I A L T O P A S K C C

L J N W O B K M L J J Y V I Z U M V D P K U W

F C G Y K X P E T J H S U C F R I E M Y S R X

Q A B O R I G I N A L U T I L G N W I Y T E K

R D E T H E R E A L M J E K T O E S T O R H W

O E N P L P C E F D D C R T T V E Y C X C C Y

M A V V H O S P I T A L U Y A A R V X R Y V Z

P D M M Q U W J G Q N W S J M R I S N A I L T

S M D K W M M H O J J P C J T Y N A U Z O F T

D N W U B O B E D S L B L X O C G T Q D V A T

W Y Y S S S Z K L P T I N S U R A N C E F P F

U V E Y O U C U Y A D V M E W V V H T K E H X

W F X G W Q H T C C O K Z J B A W D Y Q O C R

P F G R B B I K N E S F Z N A I R G W S A X X

DOMINEERING, RACIAL, SOPHISTICATED, UTERUS, CERVIX, BAWDY, ETHEREAL, OVARY, SNAIL, ADMIT, PENITENT, HYSTERECTOMY, CORRECT, RASPY, GODLY, SPACE, AIR, HOSPITAL, ABORIGINAL, DEAD, INSURANCE, WOMB, CURE

W	O	W	E	G	R	H	A	P	P	Y	H	K	D	G	G	H	K	W	H	B	K	B
R	F	T	V	N	N	W	P	S	Y	C	B	X	A	I	F	F	L	K	S	P	V	U
E	U	E	X	B	M	Q	R	P	V	G	D	P	S	P	O	O	K	Y	P	H	B	S
L	B	I	O	C	K	E	E	A	X	M	O	Y	J	R	Y	D	N	X	F	S	A	Y
A	Q	I	Z	B	E	D	G	Q	U	J	R	E	P	L	Y	U	D	G	Z	D	S	G
T	M	H	Z	J	S	Y	N	D	W	T	L	A	H	A	F	Q	O	E	E	D	K	H
I	F	S	V	S	E	R	A	E	V	C	U	X	U	E	N	C	H	A	N	T	E	D
O	C	E	L	N	D	P	N	A	U	R	E	T	H	R	A	X	O	H	Q	N	T	V
N	V	M	L	C	B	S	C	L	W	F	E	T	C	H	C	Z	D	O	Q	L	B	Y
W	G	P	H	I	T	G	Y	Q	J	G	S	G	S	R	B	A	V	U	J	A	A	Z
H	C	K	Z	A	A	Y	V	H	A	L	L	O	W	E	D	T	T	S	Y	E	L	X
I	M	A	G	I	N	A	R	Y	J	K	J	U	O	W	C	T	X	E	W	W	L	O
Y	B	K	N	B	G	F	X	N	D	E	Q	U	W	D	P	E	L	K	H	T	A	V
C	N	T	Y	U	Y	E	J	I	N	B	O	O	R	P	U	N	Q	F	Q	K	D	S
F	E	R	T	I	L	I	Z	A	T	I	O	N	H	I	L	D	M	H	N	K	U	M
W	Z	F	Y	S	W	L	C	Q	A	S	L	Q	J	H	P	N	R	A	I	S	E	N
R	L	K	X	N	U	H	H	N	N	X	D	Z	F	P	P	Z	G	F	X	S	F	S
D	D	A	S	W	E	A	T	E	R	B	S	E	P	T	X	J	E	U	Q	W	N	Z
J	S	U	R	G	E	R	Y	E	Z	F	C	C	D	E	V	G	H	Y	G	T	U	V
B	O	T	P	N	B	S	X	W	F	E	A	F	L	N	Y	T	F	V	Q	I	A	M
B	I	P	I	M	I	G	H	T	Y	R	R	P	U	A	P	O	I	K	G	W	G	V
I	H	S	E	G	A	T	G	D	P	K	E	L	J	S	P	Q	I	O	H	U	D	U
K	B	M	E	N	S	U	R	A	T	I	O	N	P	Q	E	C	Z	R	N	D	H	C

REPLY, SURGERY, URETHRA, RAISE, MIGHTY, ENCHANTED, IMAGINARY, ATTEND, SWEATER, MENSURATION, TAN, FERTILIZATION, FETCH, HOUSE, SPOOKY, HAPPY, PREGNANCY, HALLOWED, BASKETBALL, RELATION, SCARE, BUSY, TANGY

T	H	H	F	E	T	U	S	D	J	O	H	N	W	K	U	P	A	P	J	O	I	X
S	C	Y	M	N	B	O	A	S	T	M	N	L	H	P	U	E	N	V	I	S	Z	I
G	U	T	J	R	H	Q	E	N	G	W	A	N	T	S	X	L	Y	S	I	F	V	I
M	F	P	Y	U	P	M	A	B	M	B	X	U	B	L	W	V	J	F	M	T	S	E
M	I	O	B	P	V	A	C	C	I	N	E	Q	R	E	F	I	P	T	T	Y	R	X
D	Y	S	F	U	N	C	T	I	O	N	A	L	I	Y	S	S	T	U	M	P	P	J
G	C	G	H	U	P	N	V	Y	A	H	C	B	E	I	R	G	R	A	P	E	S	L
H	W	U	E	W	J	K	I	Y	G	H	N	O	F	A	Q	C	U	W	M	W	V	E
Y	V	H	I	M	T	M	X	M	N	V	M	M	A	T	C	H	W	O	R	X	N	T
I	U	V	Z	Z	D	I	Y	D	I	S	A	P	P	E	A	R	D	G	A	E	L	T
D	A	R	N	Z	L	M	H	V	N	L	D	E	L	D	P	T	W	X	J	R	V	E
U	O	A	S	D	M	R	O	P	R	Z	L	Q	X	N	M	D	M	W	Z	I	T	R
J	J	V	K	Z	P	X	Y	A	X	A	U	U	N	K	E	M	P	T	G	P	E	B
E	I	I	F	A	R	O	D	G	E	G	I	U	O	R	A	H	O	P	F	E	U	B
U	Z	H	H	G	I	J	L	C	T	R	I	T	A	U	G	Y	K	O	J	E	T	J
S	K	C	M	E	V	U	S	L	Y	E	F	E	Z	B	S	D	V	P	I	Z	L	I
J	U	J	A	G	A	X	X	A	F	E	R	L	Z	R	N	O	E	M	B	R	Y	O
K	J	U	F	G	T	Q	E	M	V	M	N	O	L	L	D	L	N	M	P	B	G	Q
J	O	R	E	S	E	N	O	N	D	E	S	C	R	I	P	T	O	B	C	X	A	S
Y	U	R	M	C	Q	T	P	O	L	N	B	K	H	Q	C	E	M	Y	S	A	X	J
G	G	Y	A	U	W	Y	K	K	X	T	P	I	H	K	S	Q	O	F	L	N	W	R
V	Q	C	L	O	A	B	S	M	O	G	G	Y	X	V	E	M	U	K	O	A	U	V
C	V	D	E	B	W	I	J	L	S	S	S	X	X	T	P	L	S	S	X	V	Q	H

MATCH, VENOMOUS, NONDESCRIPT, BOAST, CLAM, DYSFUNCTIONAL, ANTS, RUB, EGGS, BRIEF, UNKEMPT, AGREEMENT, FEMALE, SMOGGY, PRIVATE, VACCINE, GRAPE, LETTER, EMBRYO, RIPE, FETUS, DISAPPEAR, PELVIS

S	T	R	A	P	G	V	X	D	Y	C	Y	O	P	E	U	E	G	O	R	G
F	A	K	H	J	K	E	F	Q	P	M	U	K	V	C	W	U	U	E	G	D
W	Y	N	W	P	J	M	D	Y	P	H	C	Y	Q	R	H	P	A	H	L	T
Q	B	U	K	D	M	N	L	V	C	E	I	S	W	F	W	B	R	W	R	H
R	Y	Z	O	X	T	R	I	M	M	O	T	H	E	R	X	S	A	S	R	H
V	I	P	X	M	Y	G	Z	L	N	A	M	E	V	B	A	E	N	K	E	K
E	I	A	C	J	W	A	V	E	F	L	C	J	L	U	K	I	T	S	C	K
E	S	R	Y	U	O	D	U	Q	I	O	K	K	I	R	C	B	E	R	B	P
W	G	T	N	W	L	H	L	J	G	Y	R	Q	T	Y	F	R	E	R	P	C
F	I	N	A	Y	F	R	A	N	T	I	C	W	T	U	E	O	M	I	X	J
E	L	E	V	P	X	P	S	I	Q	C	O	L	L	A	R	B	Z	Q	F	P
Q	E	R	E	B	U	G	U	S	T	Y	H	O	E	A	Z	G	N	L	L	F
L	A	O	B	J	E	C	T	S	A	A	K	J	E	W	R	J	E	X	F	R
K	T	T	R	I	T	G	J	J	N	P	E	A	C	E	F	U	L	F	R	E
O	H	J	A	B	R	X	C	F	C	H	Z	J	B	F	W	S	L	E	E	Y
H	E	S	I	N	A	R	S	N	W	B	Z	T	B	Y	V	O	L	H	Q	M
A	R	S	N	I	D	J	W	X	V	U	B	R	Q	K	K	Z	Z	A	U	K
V	Z	B	Y	J	R	J	I	U	I	N	T	E	R	F	E	R	E	R	E	O
R	E	S	T	O	O	N	N	Q	X	Y	E	A	S	X	I	R	F	S	N	V
K	J	P	T	J	P	V	G	U	X	K	V	T	Q	X	F	J	I	H	T	D
H	F	T	S	N	I	N	T	E	R	E	S	T	I	N	G	T	S	F	B	L

COLLAR, SWING, MOTHER, INTERESTING, DROP, FREQUENT, STRAP, GUARANTEE, NAME, TREAT, OBJECT, BRAINY, HARSH, REST, WAVE, GUSTY, PEACEFUL, FRANTIC, LITTLE, PARTNER, LEATHER, INTERFERE, BURY

P	Z	R	L	Y	G	D	W	H	Y	O	Q	F	G	H	D	W	C
H	Z	B	R	L	Q	G	C	S	C	A	Z	F	A	I	R	A	S
Y	V	I	S	O	H	D	Z	W	O	D	V	E	T	N	U	N	V
S	O	F	P	P	E	K	Y	K	R	R	R	G	T	P	D	I	J
I	L	O	O	S	D	H	F	G	N	S	T	R	A	N	G	E	X
C	C	I	T	I	U	E	M	H	S	E	Z	U	C	Z	W	W	M
A	A	A	T	D	C	A	C	Y	W	U	G	R	H	M	W	M	C
L	N	P	E	E	A	V	W	R	A	P	A	Y	M	P	W	S	R
I	O	S	D	D	T	Y	A	M	A	Z	I	N	G	U	Q	I	Z
Z	Z	V	I	O	E	W	K	H	L	O	N	G	I	N	G	S	Z
M	E	K	L	U	D	Z	D	A	R	F	O	O	L	G	B	S	T
F	R	O	G	S	F	D	F	N	N	Q	M	T	X	N	D	U	C
L	A	V	I	S	H	Z	X	D	W	N	E	L	R	P	O	P	F
S	L	E	R	E	C	T	L	S	N	A	M	P	W	E	C	P	W
B	M	L	E	C	S	M	R	O	O	Q	O	O	M	T	T	O	N
A	V	B	V	F	F	P	P	M	E	Q	R	U	L	S	O	S	E
Q	D	Y	H	B	F	G	V	E	D	I	Y	R	J	Y	R	E	N
T	P	U	L	E	E	K	Z	P	Q	P	O	E	Y	Z	S	R	H

LAVISH, FOOL, CORN, SPOTTED, HEAVY, WRAP, POUR, HANDSOME, ERECT, AMAZING, LONGING, LOPSIDED, STRANGE, ATTACH, SUPPOSE, DOCTORS, MEMORY, PHYSICAL, FAIR, EDUCATED, VOLCANO, PETS, FROGS

Q	N	F	A	I	T	H	F	U	L	J	I	I	S	H	C	H	K	Z	H
H	L	T	J	Z	A	T	D	R	Y	K	Z	E	F	J	H	F	E	T	H
I	L	S	A	G	T	E	F	F	I	C	I	E	N	T	I	R	T	R	L
B	L	U	S	H	M	V	Q	Z	S	C	Q	Q	R	O	E	D	A	V	R
O	Z	F	U	F	D	Y	U	S	J	B	E	K	Y	L	F	B	A	B	Y
D	Y	G	N	R	U	F	J	O	C	Z	S	G	F	U	I	T	R	E	Z
D	S	S	U	Y	G	S	H	O	E	E	D	I	Q	S	U	H	Q	Z	W
Y	X	H	M	Q	W	O	G	U	B	X	U	C	X	F	E	U	B	Z	L
Q	U	A	R	T	E	R	R	A	F	Z	Y	Q	S	O	R	N	R	Z	T
J	W	R	O	N	G	M	A	A	G	B	I	U	T	Z	M	D	E	T	V
K	C	L	U	O	J	O	N	J	T	B	G	E	R	T	K	E	S	C	G
B	W	O	N	E	W	T	D	E	S	O	O	E	E	W	V	R	C	Y	T
V	E	Z	H	P	U	I	I	F	C	R	V	N	T	L	N	I	U	V	S
X	L	M	A	R	B	O	O	L	V	R	E	N	C	Z	F	N	E	E	C
G	L	T	R	A	E	N	S	K	L	O	R	Y	H	C	L	G	I	K	I
R	-	L	M	Z	L	L	E	L	U	W	N	T	S	T	E	W	X	L	S
Q	O	A	Z	Z	A	E	N	M	V	D	O	R	E	V	Q	M	J	W	S
B	F	Y	C	Y	G	S	J	R	H	W	R	L	H	G	T	W	P	V	O
Z	F	T	P	V	G	S	B	F	R	R	A	D	I	A	T	E	W	C	R
W	F	E	I	I	M	J	H	J	T	U	Y	H	L	Z	A	G	E	Q	S

FAITHFUL, SHOE, QUEEN, THUNDERING, CHIEF, GOVERNOR, QUARTER, MOTIONLESS, SCISSORS, EFFICIENT, BABY, ONE, WRONG, BLUSH, GRANDIOSE, WELL-OFF, DRY, ODD, STRETCH, STEW, BORROW, RESCUE, RADIATE

U	D	E	B	W	Z	T	I	X	F	P	M	K	L	B	Y	U	G	X	T	C
D	U	S	T	Y	P	I	O	B	A	B	Q	F	F	A	S	S	C	J	J	S
W	H	S	O	O	Q	C	H	C	J	Y	B	L	P	Q	K	P	D	M	V	J
M	O	N	D	V	P	K	S	J	Y	Y	Y	K	F	I	W	Q	J	S	C	P
I	U	P	R	I	V	E	R	Q	G	J	F	F	K	M	E	Z	K	S	T	Y
D	S	J	F	P	I	T	K	P	X	Z	C	J	E	O	X	E	L	Y	T	V
J	F	S	T	U	P	I	D	C	T	R	U	L	E	L	P	C	P	F	O	J
F	P	B	B	O	T	Y	A	F	T	E	R	M	A	T	H	T	P	T	V	O
J	T	A	O	D	H	V	T	E	F	F	I	C	A	C	I	O	U	S	M	Y
R	O	T	T	S	R	Y	G	G	S	L	Z	P	W	W	T	R	N	L	C	O
X	U	H	T	L	O	O	K	A	J	E	U	Z	G	R	P	L	C	M	M	U
N	C	E	L	H	A	K	R	R	P	C	Y	C	M	B	O	R	H	C	S	S
M	H	N	E	T	T	W	A	Y	A	T	C	M	Z	V	T	A	P	Y	L	S
X	V	J	B	Q	J	Z	V	A	S	I	N	J	U	R	E	E	E	F	E	J
I	E	K	Z	S	F	J	T	Q	S	G	V	J	M	M	N	U	R	E	E	O
C	H	E	M	I	C	A	L	T	E	U	W	P	U	D	O	M	F	J	T	Z
R	E	L	X	M	B	X	I	G	N	E	G	I	G	W	Y	L	E	O	Y	G
B	M	Z	Z	W	O	L	C	K	G	I	G	Y	Q	D	W	H	C	M	F	X
R	J	G	I	O	X	H	K	L	E	Z	F	N	N	H	M	J	T	L	T	G
E	Y	W	Q	E	V	W	V	V	R	S	B	Y	L	B	A	L	A	N	C	E
M	G	O	Q	R	Q	U	U	T	P	Q	T	C	U	T	D	L	A	U	A	H

SLEET, TOUCH, POT, CHEMICAL, JOYOUS, BALANCE, STUPID, TICKET, REFLECT, EFFICACIOUS, PERFECT, BATHE, AFTERMATH, THROAT, PASSENGER, INJURE, BOTTLE, LOOK, RIVER, MUG, CUT, WAY, DUSTY

Z	V	G	M	L	B	P	Z	W	T	F	I	T	P	J	D	W	Y	N	U
Q	P	Q	G	V	S	I	A	I	S	Z	M	P	R	O	F	I	T	G	Z
M	W	K	I	Q	M	P	G	N	R	W	P	W	F	L	O	W	E	R	Y
N	Q	S	Y	J	W	E	P	D	Z	X	R	B	A	E	L	I	T	E	H
O	B	T	S	N	T	U	X	O	G	S	E	R	E	K	B	O	I	X	Y
V	D	N	G	D	C	J	C	W	K	K	S	W	U	S	K	I	N	D	T
H	A	D	S	T	U	B	L	O	O	D	S	X	W	V	G	P	B	H	J
Q	R	C	C	G	J	I	T	T	E	R	Y	X	Y	G	U	N	C	E	L
S	U	U	R	L	C	O	M	M	I	T	T	E	E	Q	A	K	N	M	R
Y	T	V	I	S	R	K	C	Y	J	W	M	U	D	Y	V	J	L	B	A
M	A	D	B	X	V	B	U	B	O	R	I	N	G	T	V	U	H	B	P
C	S	V	B	R	W	L	P	W	J	U	G	G	L	E	H	O	U	Z	J
G	T	C	L	I	M	O	H	X	A	F	R	A	I	D	K	S	C	N	H
A	E	I	E	A	R	I	T	H	M	E	T	I	C	O	W	S	H	E	U
L	L	P	I	L	R	T	X	P	A	R	C	E	L	V	X	I	I	Q	N
C	E	Z	R	B	Q	I	G	X	M	A	R	K	E	T	R	F	L	W	I
J	S	B	L	U	E	-	E	Y	E	D	G	R	I	Y	K	I	Y	W	T
V	S	O	A	B	Z	K	Y	X	Z	W	D	E	J	F	P	E	V	T	I
W	K	E	P	R	A	C	T	I	C	E	C	T	V	E	W	D	E	O	A
J	E	I	M	Z	W	A	T	C	H	Q	R	C	Q	V	T	Q	B	T	S

PARCEL, JITTERY, BORING, PIPE, JUGGLE, PROFIT, MARKET, OSSIFIED, IMPRESS, SCRIBBLE, BLOOD, FLOWERY, SKIN, ARITHMETIC, COMMITTEE, AFRAID, PRACTICE, BLUE-EYED, TASTELESS, WATCH, WINDOW, UNIT, ELITE

B	H	E	Z	H	I	F	R	V	K	R	M	N	Z	G	V	F	O	H	E	G
J	W	Z	K	I	B	F	L	Y	I	N	G	K	N	M	X	X	S	A	L	S
Z	C	L	O	N	G	-	T	E	R	M	W	A	X	G	I	Q	G	A	O	F
R	X	P	G	O	B	S	E	R	V	A	T	I	O	N	S	U	L	Y	M	I
Q	R	O	Z	T	M	E	I	M	I	N	O	R	N	Z	A	E	Q	A	J	H
Y	E	P	P	R	S	S	H	U	G	G	H	J	X	H	T	T	S	P	T	Z
U	C	E	H	C	W	O	F	Y	T	A	P	P	E	A	R	E	Q	G	H	B
V	O	N	C	S	C	L	E	V	E	L	A	K	S	I	Q	V	B	C	I	L
X	R	A	R	G	U	E	G	U	C	W	X	G	A	F	G	F	P	A	R	E
Z	D	W	S	X	P	D	S	A	N	J	O	M	V	Q	M	F	M	L	S	R
T	N	S	U	I	N	C	Z	K	O	A	L	O	O	D	I	Q	D	C	T	C
R	Q	N	T	A	R	T	N	V	R	R	E	U	R	U	C	B	H	U	Y	P
A	J	J	K	D	U	G	Y	P	T	M	A	N	Y	S	E	R	N	L	T	B
D	X	I	T	L	G	F	R	G	H	G	Z	T	Z	I	Z	U	A	A	W	V
E	A	K	R	P	I	S	A	K	A	M	E	A	K	S	N	H	X	T	L	O
P	P	K	E	J	D	G	Z	K	F	L	U	I	I	T	J	A	V	E	S	B
I	K	F	P	H	D	O	K	F	I	F	S	N	M	E	E	Q	T	O	Q	P
B	C	A	E	A	Y	S	D	M	T	B	G	O	P	R	T	P	F	D	M	L
F	X	S	A	U	R	A	B	B	I	T	S	U	J	S	N	Y	F	T	X	J
V	A	T	T	N	O	H	E	Q	D	J	M	S	H	O	V	H	U	I	W	J
W	Z	Y	N	T	W	Y	Q	K	S	Y	P	A	V	T	U	Z	O	I	J	I

SAVORY, REPEAT, ARGUE, TART, LYING, MINOR, CALCULATE, MOUNTAINOUS, APPEAR, LONG-TERM, THIRSTY, TRADE, SISTERS, HUG, OBSERVATION, RECORD, MICE, HAUNT, FAST, RABBITS, GIDDY, NORTH, LEVEL

X	A	N	V	Y	N	S	Y	R	T	F	D	Y	P	I	C	T	U	R	E	X	V	N
H	L	V	D	I	V	B	U	A	U	K	W	P	O	E	J	D	A	M	B	R	Z	S
N	Q	U	I	Y	L	T	R	I	L	A	R	Q	F	H	W	X	B	F	T	I	S	L
W	S	G	S	D	L	D	B	Z	R	U	D	L	I	Z	F	B	Y	L	G	J	L	L
B	K	A	I	G	E	Y	C	F	K	G	I	N	F	L	E	H	Y	R	E	G	L	D
U	B	V	L	P	E	Y	C	G	A	H	M	L	L	N	Z	Y	G	D	T	V	F	B
O	S	R	L	A	Q	U	A	T	I	C	E	J	M	R	Q	Y	E	U	T	F	S	M
P	Q	T	U	J	S	U	R	P	R	I	S	E	C	A	U	S	N	L	V	I	F	A
P	T	T	S	A	F	V	D	X	C	U	W	P	Y	P	E	N	E	L	C	N	X	U
Y	R	K	I	I	F	S	O	D	P	M	S	R	Z	I	L	G	R	G	S	O	U	L
R	E	H	O	C	Z	E	V	X	A	S	U	F	Q	D	N	P	G	T	T	H	A	S
G	I	G	N	Q	Q	B	E	L	I	M	I	T	F	X	K	F	E	V	R	L	A	M
L	Y	D	E	G	K	U	N	D	R	E	S	S	A	Y	R	H	T	H	A	W	C	E
R	X	B	D	O	H	W	P	H	J	W	X	L	N	U	A	R	I	Z	I	F	T	L
D	A	A	D	A	C	R	I	D	R	S	T	A	B	D	K	L	C	W	G	C	I	L
R	J	Z	F	A	C	P	I	W	L	R	M	U	F	N	R	D	B	K	H	H	V	U
B	F	E	S	Z	Y	I	Z	T	D	T	I	G	A	A	T	V	V	H	T	F	I	N
U	Q	B	B	B	N	C	M	H	M	Z	T	H	B	D	B	J	S	M	E	A	T	W
U	U	D	S	K	I	A	X	Y	P	R	E	A	U	R	U	L	E	B	O	A	Y	E
T	M	L	C	D	C	Y	D	G	E	V	P	B	H	I	L	L	-	F	A	T	E	D
K	V	C	U	A	A	U	C	R	N	S	P	L	J	C	F	P	Y	J	Y	W	N	I
W	T	P	T	S	L	N	Q	G	K	G	M	E	P	Z	L	B	P	O	W	D	E	R
F	H	Y	H	M	Y	E	F	Q	O	C	O	S	I	W	B	U	O	H	E	F	C	J

STRAIGHT, CYNICAL, PEN, DIME, DISILLUSIONED, SURPRISE, ILL-FATED, POWDER, DULL, LIMIT, UNDRESS, LAUGHABLE, ENERGETIC, OVEN, PICTURE, AQUATIC, RULE, ACTIVITY, MEAT, SMELL, PICAYUNE, RAPID, ACRID

WORD SCRAMBLE

hitosyr = _______________	rnoesa = _______________	daln = _______________
pxiealn = _______________	intnoa = _______________	lsea = _______________
eesceh = _______________	uennev = _______________	veableetg = _______________
ayre = _______________	oitudrnce = _______________	ykawc = _______________
tconolr = _______________	ebtlat = _______________	oacrcwrse = _______________
ergua = _______________	needticro = _______________	irentims = _______________
pehlass = _______________	ogdelenkw = _______________	euisrldio = _______________
seerag = _______________	yeplr = _______________	tccciuns = _______________
ldrcenhi = _______________	ekrcw = _______________	vdeser = _______________
skdi = _______________	ntteibfig = _______________	iep = _______________
thgsatir = _______________	aghsyg = _______________	roeshs = _______________
rewi = _______________	owt = _______________	ptmarroey = _______________
atehncig = _______________	aoalisflcu = _______________	lsgliseut = _______________
eto = _______________	rbttee = _______________	helsisf = _______________
encnait = _______________	ifturicust = _______________	gnbiondua = _______________
alpi = _______________	ecrcnno = _______________	iytn = _______________
istan = _______________	vryao = _______________	bmbo = _______________
likae = _______________	hripwse = _______________	dewrra = _______________
ntua = _______________	cbul = _______________	tne = _______________
testyoerdpe = _______________	frfoe = _______________	leohsmse = _______________
drtees = _______________	ores = _______________	trsa = _______________
ouepdrecr = _______________	ikle = _______________	irdet = _______________
eafc = _______________	eeatld = _______________	hesoanmd = _______________
gmu = _______________	yersrug = _______________	eagadm = _______________
eaelgld = _______________	spudnse = _______________	poilte = _______________
dehya = _______________	fieecr = _______________	ggdeaj = _______________
mxeid = _______________	mesyel = _______________	rdwaer = _______________
aecnhg = _______________	kieb = _______________	

bdyaw = _______________	zppiy = _______________	nnitvnoie = _______________
eeosvbr = _______________	mo-dilferiln = _______________	eaifntinmcg = _______________
bssel = _______________	robe = _______________	ahignlt = _______________
esav = _______________	nhdas = _______________	ynarg = _______________
dodris = _______________	elgrgwi = _______________	arepg = _______________
aesm = _______________	vcrae = _______________	coefif = _______________
styud = _______________	rcko = _______________	jciyu = _______________
nrdik = _______________	atmse = _______________	xceept = _______________
atbcje = _______________	hwso = _______________	llyhci = _______________
jaar = _______________	wedi = _______________	actmh = _______________
dadfe = _______________	etsb = _______________	erme = _______________
ipt = _______________	llki = _______________	emab = _______________
asbvieu = _______________	accho = _______________	ntslei = _______________
roucc = _______________	ehtarg = _______________	snirg = _______________
guesiosntg = _______________	yto = _______________	rolco = _______________
aenubl = _______________	dgstseuid = _______________	aoihsctirl = _______________
asnild = _______________	egsuqorte = _______________	ohpsli = _______________
gteer = _______________	teha = _______________	gdo = _______________
cluoro = _______________	uryfr = _______________	ujcie = _______________
ioslfho = _______________	auermt = _______________	tooba = _______________
fhllyejis = _______________	eratbh = _______________	ift = _______________
tdaapbeal = _______________	rpiotd = _______________	tpslan = _______________
lsdopdei = _______________	nlnei = _______________	lsseoensi = _______________
aretspea = _______________	ciceli = _______________	evlog = _______________
iprd = _______________	eownm = _______________	refgila = _______________
eaulngga = _______________	lpaec = _______________	eodrrc = _______________
shpi = _______________	ckud = _______________	ipcslea = _______________
nslsai = _______________	osgd = _______________	

ptol = _______________	ethra = _______________	riyalaw = _______________
crtik = _______________	alfl = _______________	eirdma = _______________
mtea = _______________	csennecantid = _______________	ogeurthtfaht = _______________
lgael = _______________	apss = _______________	hstor = _______________
rwlngiseet = _______________	ennetmi = _______________	rkacecr = _______________
uler = _______________	heom = _______________	pli = _______________
mreobdo = _______________	nilap = _______________	owdo = _______________
ttor = _______________	add = _______________	cnctnoe = _______________
maen = _______________	wlla = _______________	nsilmig = _______________
ddleum = _______________	exlmcop = _______________	aetr = _______________
mnsyaelohd = _______________	defa = _______________	chnrab = _______________
laacir = _______________	xfi = _______________	rmteip = _______________
usceex = _______________	hhubotorts = _______________	etderesd = _______________
ancarpimo = _______________	kyic = _______________	terbeha = _______________
eisncce = _______________	koej = _______________	smeok = _______________
ricep = _______________	lelagaubh = _______________	rgean = _______________
urby = _______________	reeientgc = _______________	lpci = _______________
opiposte = _______________	ookc = _______________	byburg = _______________
ymtsse = _______________	tlsi = _______________	hdaea = _______________
lbsle = _______________	edsi = _______________	snece = _______________
jial = _______________	fruaegcl = _______________	niasb = _______________
mayginiar = _______________	wihge = _______________	cmlia = _______________
tsraw = _______________	ttseacr = _______________	uhtom = _______________
tsecoinel = _______________	iqursrle = _______________	ucbntssea = _______________
iehfc = _______________	eky = _______________	eoudstrvnua = _______________
needrabsuil = _______________	ncsosit = _______________	ebluod = _______________
ooz = _______________	eclnu = _______________	uacatmito = _______________
wlohdela = _______________	rusga = _______________	

kyeo = _______________	uemngtar = _______________	sviroit = _______________
fspreou = _______________	predwo = _______________	cerdeep = _______________
erutfu = _______________	eesnt = _______________	bnguslhi = _______________
ssderpi = _______________	ilrg = _______________	tsrbu = _______________
tro = _______________	xaaicoitm = _______________	rhtcsac = _______________
kdscu = _______________	taseg = _______________	neam = _______________
irbno = _______________	wienressld = _______________	zpipre = _______________
ofas = _______________	aotrth = _______________	xnuosoi = _______________
bicrk = _______________	usohied = _______________	hibtaual = _______________
tbrgih = _______________	hiegt = _______________	abgcbea = _______________
aner = _______________	rulc = _______________	htwac = _______________
ulbsh = _______________	ganh = _______________	ettpamt = _______________
eovrdarte = _______________	c ohda = _______________	llsma = _______________
rnya = _______________	orfm = _______________	saetuqeust = _______________
dod = _______________	iepyrc = _______________	nenuacno = _______________
efhrs = _______________	rgni = _______________	ahfolsidd-eno = _______________
tba = _______________	gsons = _______________	rpesu = _______________
unt = _______________	feowovrl = _______________	bvlelaaai = _______________
liacdiascakal = _______________	omwr = _______________	npla = _______________
ancrve = _______________	ocsrch = _______________	ldbea = _______________
irsarotnm = _______________	ehos = _______________	htgouht = _______________
nlidb = _______________	aethd = _______________	tecdte = _______________
lcpien = _______________	aerusq = _______________	ngriomn = _______________
omseonru = _______________	lbtea = _______________	htgyim = _______________
cokl = _______________	ftnenasu = _______________	triks = _______________
tteeh = _______________	nsoe = _______________	rwnob = _______________
eulf = _______________	cavesnente = _______________	cnrow = _______________
tffcee = _______________	ssutrero = _______________	

oidniuiss = _______________	titnem = _______________	tqkiescu = _______________
lufl = _______________	plsmeiu = _______________	grvgiine = _______________
okocr = _______________	mjntadsteu = _______________	pdsoei = _______________
naeemtrtt = _______________	wretahe = _______________	ktsea = _______________
mresmu = _______________	terecilc = _______________	uhcog = _______________
tlme = _______________	avlue = _______________	cnneontoic = _______________
ysk = _______________	pcihn = _______________	syot = _______________
arrcy = _______________	thscti = _______________	phees = _______________
ctas = _______________	rsiceeex = _______________	d-nhfdor-iat = _______________
ulqit = _______________	asepnxoin = _______________	cynkuh = _______________
ntegmnevro = _______________	eknfi = _______________	snefsco = _______________
nliactglacu = _______________	tlbo = _______________	asw = _______________
oeynh = _______________	lgdo = _______________	stgrane = _______________
tepeti = _______________	inwwdo = _______________	ianr = _______________
itck = _______________	ddaeeeft = _______________	esselus = _______________
osuseh = _______________	nnecmddoe = _______________	cyr = _______________
nlaufgi = _______________	eumitn = _______________	libo = _______________
osncucleniiv = _______________	anudatnb = _______________	xfdie = _______________
mnoo = _______________	tecer = _______________	arenewdur = _______________
lsani = _______________	rstetine = _______________	ptar = _______________
ddea = _______________	pigr = _______________	ogayve = _______________
ofto = _______________	ahbt = _______________	rtecpes = _______________
obmser = _______________	nwie = _______________	pttem = _______________
ctkis = _______________	hnit = _______________	spta = _______________
odirncse = _______________	mreci = _______________	ydslftcninoua = _______________
elbla = _______________	ralpyt = _______________	vlao = _______________
uhormuso = _______________	auiirstlp = _______________	elfs = _______________
pesmoliibs = _______________	eejlw = _______________	

Solutions

hitosyr	=	history	rnoesa	=	reason	daln	=	land
pxiealn	=	explain	intnoa	=	nation	lsea	=	seal
eesceh	=	cheese	uennev	=	uneven	veableetg	=	vegetable
ayre	=	year	oitudrnce	=	introduce	ykawc	=	wacky
tconolr	=	control	ebtlat	=	battle	oacrcwrse	=	scarecrow
ergua	=	argue	needticro	=	recondite	irentims	=	minister
pehlass	=	hapless	ogdelenkw	=	knowledge	euisrldio	=	delirious
seerag	=	grease	yeplr	=	reply	tccciuns	=	succinct
ldrcenhi	=	children	ekrcw	=	wreck	vdeser	=	versed
skdi	=	kids	ntteibfig	=	befitting	iep	=	pie
thgsatir	=	straight	aghsyg	=	shaggy	roeshs	=	horses
rewi	=	wire	owt	=	two	ptmarroey	=	temporary
atehncig	=	teaching	aoalisflcu	=	fallacious	lsgliseut	=	guiltless
eto	=	toe	rbttee	=	better	helsisf	=	selfish
encnait	=	ancient	ifturicust	=	futuristic	gnbiondua	=	abounding
alpi	=	pail	ecrcnno	=	concern	iytn	=	tiny
istan	=	stain	vryao	=	ovary	bmbo	=	bomb
likae	=	alike	hripwse	=	whisper	dewrra	=	drawer
ntua	=	aunt	cbul	=	club	tne	=	ten
testyoerdpe	=	stereotyped	frfoe	=	offer	leohsmse	=	homeless
drtees	=	desert	ores	=	rose	trsa	=	star
ouepdrecr	=	reproduce	ikle	=	like	irdet	=	tired
eafc	=	face	eeatld	=	elated	hesoanmd	=	handsome
gmu	=	mug	yersrug	=	surgery	eagadm	=	damage
eaelgld	=	alleged	spudnse	=	suspend	poilte	=	polite
dehya	=	heady	fieecr	=	fierce	ggdeaj	=	jagged
mxeid	=	mixed	mesyel	=	seemly	rdwaer	=	reward
aecnhg	=	change	kieb	=	bike			

bdyaw	=	bawdy	zppiy	=	zippy	nnitvnoie	=	invention
eeosvbr	=	observe	mo-dilferiln	=	ill-informed	eaifntinmcg	=	magnificent
bssel	=	bless	robe	=	bore	ahignlt	=	halting
esav	=	save	nhdas	=	hands	ynarg	=	angry
dodris	=	sordid	elgrgwi	=	wriggle	arepg	=	grape
aesm	=	same	vcrae	=	carve	coefif	=	office
styud	=	dusty	rcko	=	rock	jciyu	=	juicy
nrdik	=	drink	atmse	=	steam	xceept	=	expect
atbcje	=	abject	hwso	=	show	llyhci	=	chilly
jaar	=	ajar	wedi	=	wide	actmh	=	match
dadfe	=	faded	etsb	=	best	erme	=	mere
ipt	=	tip	llki	=	kill	emab	=	beam
asbvieu	=	abusive	accho	=	coach	ntslei	=	listen
roucc	=	occur	ehtarg	=	gather	snirg	=	rings
guesiosntg	=	suggestion	yto	=	toy	rolco	=	color
aenubl	=	unable	dgstseuid	=	disgusted	aoihsctirl	=	historical
asnild	=	island	egsuqorte	=	grotesque	ohpsli	=	polish
gteer	=	greet	teha	=	hate	gdo	=	dog
cluoro	=	colour	uryfr	=	furry	ujcie	=	juice
ioslfho	=	foolish	auermt	=	mature	tooba	=	taboo
fhllyejis	=	jellyfish	eratbh	=	breath	ift	=	fit
tdaapbeal	=	adaptable	rpiotd	=	torpid	tpslan	=	plants
lsdopdei	=	lopsided	nlnei	=	linen	lsseoensi	=	noiseless
aretspea	=	separate	ciceli	=	icicle	evlog	=	glove
iprd	=	drip	eownm	=	women	refgila	=	fragile
eaulngga	=	language	lpaec	=	place	eodrrc	=	record
shpi	=	ship	ckud	=	duck	ipcslea	=	special
nslsai	=	snails	osgd	=	dogs			

ptol	=	plot	ethra	=	earth	riyalaw	=	railway
crtik	=	trick	alfl	=	fall	eirdma	=	admire
mtea	=	meat	csennecantid	=	incandescent	ogeurthtfaht	=	afterthought
lgael	=	legal	apss	=	pass	hstor	=	short
rwlngiseet	=	sweltering	ennetmi	=	eminent	rkacecr	=	cracker
uler	=	rule	heom	=	home	pli	=	lip
mreobdo	=	bedroom	nilap	=	plain	owdo	=	wood
ttor	=	trot	add	=	dad	cnctnoe	=	connect
maen	=	name	wlla	=	wall	nsilmig	=	smiling
ddleum	=	muddle	exlmcop	=	complex	aetr	=	rate
mnsyaelohd	=	handsomely	defa	=	fade	chnrab	=	branch
laacir	=	racial	xfi	=	fix	rmteip	=	permit
usceex	=	excuse	hhubotorts	=	toothbrush	etderesd	=	deserted
ancarpimo	=	panoramic	kyic	=	icky	terbeha	=	breathe
eisncce	=	science	koej	=	joke	smeok	=	smoke
ricep	=	price	lelagaubh	=	laughable	rgean	=	range
urby	=	bury	reeientgc	=	energetic	lpci	=	clip
opiposte	=	opposite	ookc	=	cook	byburg	=	grubby
ymtsse	=	system	tlsi	=	list	hdaea	=	ahead
lbsle	=	bells	edsi	=	side	snece	=	scene
jial	=	jail	fruaegcl	=	graceful	niasb	=	basin
mayginiar	=	imaginary	wihge	=	weigh	cmlia	=	claim
tsraw	=	straw	ttseacr	=	scatter	uhtom	=	mouth
tsecoinel	=	selection	iqursrle	=	squirrel	ucbntssea	=	substance
iehfc	=	chief	eky	=	key	eoudstrvnua	=	adventurous
needrabsuil	=	undesirable	ncsosit	=	consist	ebluod	=	double
ooz	=	zoo	eclnu	=	uncle	uacatmito	=	automatic
wlohdela	=	hallowed	rusga	=	sugar			

kyeo	=	yoke	uemngtar	=	argument	sviroit	=	visitor
fspreou	=	profuse	predwo	=	powder	cerdeep	=	precede
erutfu	=	future	eesnt	=	tense	bnguslhi	=	blushing
ssderpi	=	spiders	ilrg	=	girl	tsrbu	=	burst
tro	=	rot	xaaicoitm	=	axiomatic	rhtcsac	=	scratch
kdscu	=	ducks	taseg	=	stage	neam	=	mean
irbno	=	robin	wienressld	=	wilderness	zpipre	=	zipper
ofas	=	sofa	aotrth	=	throat	xnuosoi	=	noxious
bicrk	=	brick	usohied	=	hideous	hibtaual	=	habitual
tbrgih	=	bright	hiegt	=	eight	abgcbea	=	cabbage
aner	=	earn	rulc	=	curl	htwac	=	watch
ulbsh	=	blush	ganh	=	hang	ettpamt	=	attempt
eovrdarte	=	overrated	c ohda	=	ad hoc	llsma	=	small
rnya	=	yarn	orfm	=	form	saetuqeust	=	statuesque
dod	=	odd	iepyrc	=	pricey	nenuacno	=	announce
efhrs	=	fresh	rgni	=	ring	ahfolsidd-eno	=	old-fashioned
tba	=	bat	gsons	=	songs	rpesu	=	super
unt	=	nut	feowovrl	=	overflow	bvlelaaai	=	available
liacdiascakal	=	lackadaisical	omwr	=	worm	npla	=	plan
ancrve	=	craven	ocsrch	=	scorch	ldbea	=	blade
irsarotnm	=	rainstorm	ehos	=	hose	htgouht	=	thought
nlidb	=	blind	aethd	=	death	tecdte	=	detect
lcpien	=	pencil	aerusq	=	square	ngriomn	=	morning
omseonru	=	enormous	lbtea	=	table	htgyim	=	mighty
cokl	=	lock	ftnenasu	=	unfasten	triks	=	skirt
tteeh	=	teeth	nsoe	=	nose	rwnob	=	brown
eulf	=	fuel	cavesnente	=	evanescent	cnrow	=	crown
tffcee	=	effect	ssutrero	=	trousers			

oidniuiss	=	insidious	titnem	=	mitten	tqkiescu	=	quickest
lufl	=	full	plsmeiu	=	impulse	grvgiine	=	grieving
okocr	=	crook	mjntadsteu	=	adjustment	pdsoei	=	poised
naeemtrtt	=	treatment	wretahe	=	weather	ktsea	=	skate
mresmu	=	summer	terecilc	=	electric	uhcog	=	cough
tlme	=	melt	avlue	=	value	cnneontoic	=	connection
ysk	=	sky	pcihn	=	pinch	syot	=	toys
arrcy	=	carry	thscti	=	stitch	phees	=	sheep
ctas	=	cats	rsiceeex	=	exercise	d-nhfdor-iat	=	hard-to-find
ulqit	=	quilt	asepnxoin	=	expansion	cynkuh	=	chunky
ntegmnevro	=	government	eknfi	=	knife	snefsco	=	confess
nliactglacu	=	calculating	tlbo	=	blot	asw	=	saw
oeynh	=	honey	lgdo	=	gold	stgrane	=	strange
tepeti	=	petite	inwwdo	=	window	ianr	=	rain
itck	=	tick	ddaeeeft	=	defeated	esselus	=	useless
osuseh	=	houses	nnecmddoe	=	condemned	cyr	=	cry
nlaufgi	=	gainful	eumitn	=	minute	libo	=	boil
osncucleniiv	=	inconclusive	anudatnb	=	abundant	xfdie	=	fixed
mnoo	=	moon	tecer	=	erect	arenewdur	=	underwear
lsani	=	snail	rstetine	=	interest	ptar	=	part
ddea	=	dead	pigr	=	grip	ogayve	=	voyage
ofto	=	foot	ahbt	=	bath	rtecpes	=	respect
obmser	=	somber	nwie	=	wine	pttem	=	tempt
ctkis	=	stick	hnit	=	thin	spta	=	past
odirncse	=	consider	mreci	=	crime	ydslftcninoua	=	dysfunctional
elbla	=	label	ralpyt	=	paltry	vlao	=	oval
uhormuso	=	humorous	auiirstlp	=	spiritual	elfs	=	self
pesmoliibs	=	impossible	eejlw	=	jewel			

Made in the USA
Columbia, SC
10 February 2025

53663331R00059

GREY CUP GLORY!

The Edmonton Eskimos' 2003 Championship Season

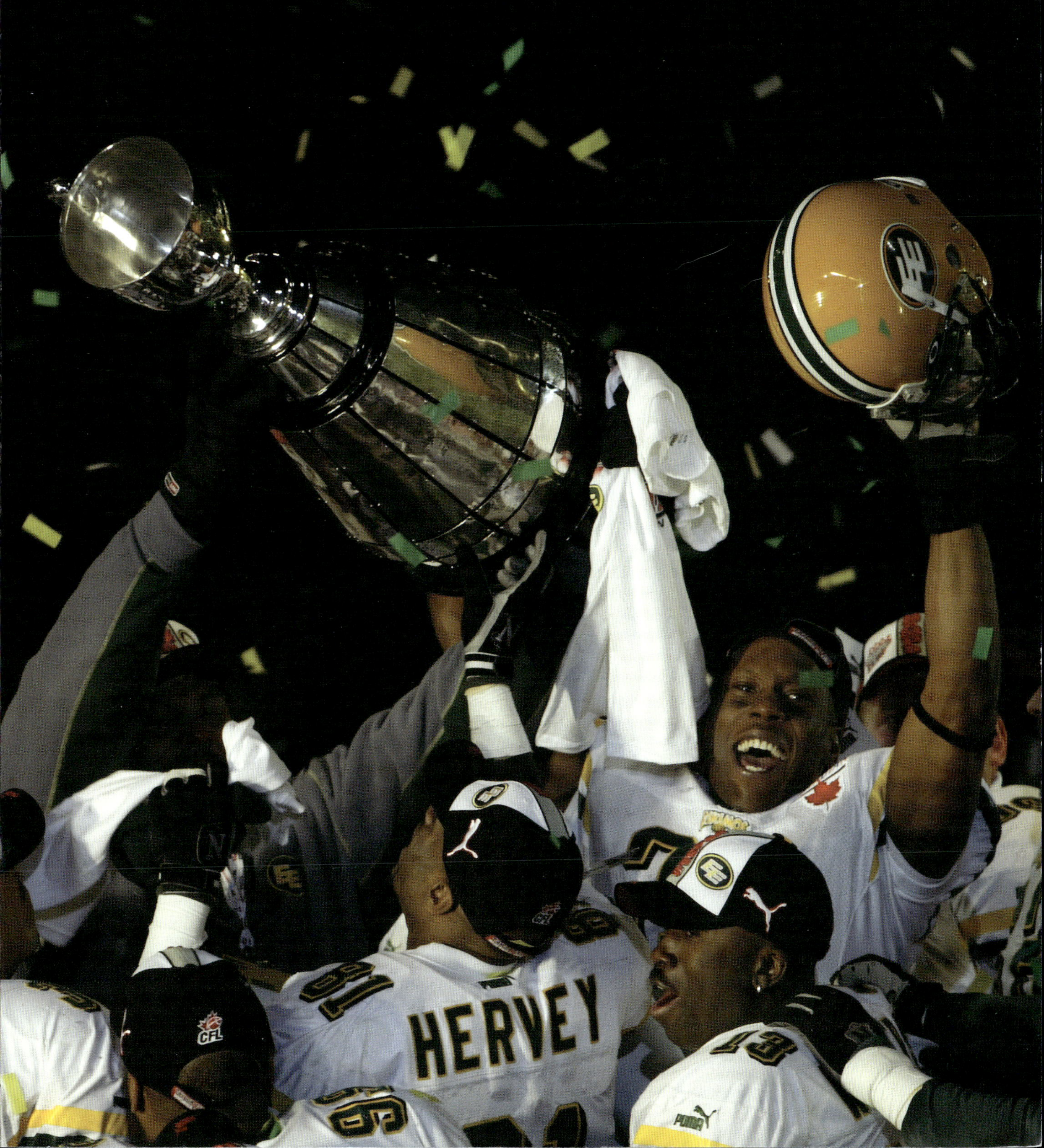

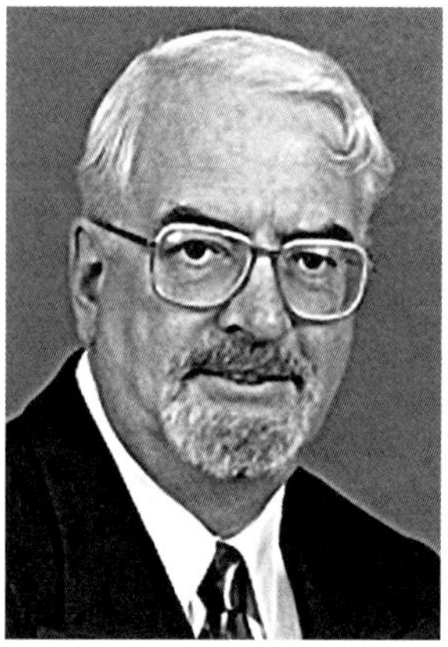

About the Author

A native of Regina, where he worked for the Roughriders as a teenager and later covered the team for United Press International, Graham Kelly has been the Canadian Football League columnist for the *Medicine Hat News* since 1972, covering 29 Grey Cups in the process. In 1999, Johnson Gorman Publishers released his first best-selling book *The Grey Cup: A History*. In 2001, Harper Collins published *Green Grit: The Story of the Saskatchewan Roughriders*.

Graham Kelly was inducted into the Canadian Football League Hall of Fame, Media Division, in November 2002.

Dedicated to the Edmonton Eskimos, past and present, and to the City of Champions.

GREY CUP GLORY!

The Edmonton Eskimos' 2003 Championship Season

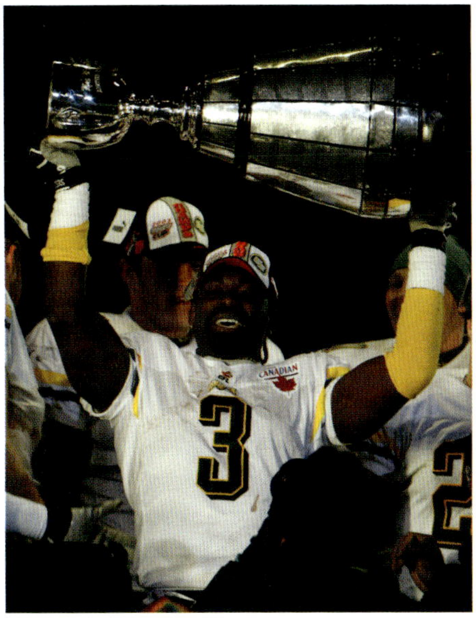

Graham Kelly

Photography by

Dale MacMillan

Johnson Gorman Publishers

The Publishers
Johnson Gorman Publishers
Calgary Alberta
www.jgbooks.com

Credits
Photography courtesy of Dale MacMillan.
Cover and text design by Full Court Press.
Special thanks to John Chaput for editorial assistance.
Printed and bound in Canada by ITS Design & Printing Inc. for Johnson Gorman Publishers.

Acknowledgments
Financial assistance provided by the Alberta Foundation for the Arts, a beneficiary of the Lottery Fund of the Government of Alberta.

COMMITTED TO THE DEVELOPMENT OF CULTURE AND THE ARTS

5 4 3 2 1

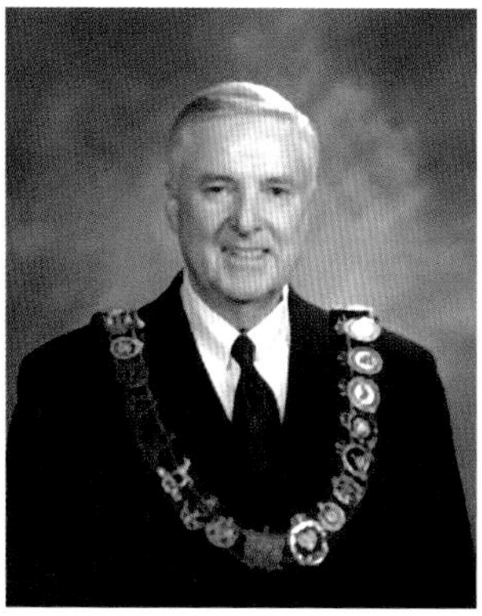

Message from His Worship Mayor Bill Smith

It is my great pleasure to support Graham Kelly's recent book, *Grey Cup Glory: The Edmonton Eskimos 2003 Championship Season*. It takes dedication, perseverance and talent to become a writer, and Graham has all of that and more.

This book is testimony to writing excellence and reflects your talents as an accomplished author and supporter of Canadian football.

On behalf of City Council and the citizens of Edmonton, I salute your outstanding contributions. We are honoured to have a leading Canadian author residing in our Province. Thank you for bringing this most deserved recognition to our beloved Edmonton Eskimos.

Yours truly,

Bill Smith
Mayor

EDMONTON ESKIMO'S 2003 WESTERN ALL-STARS

Offense

MIKE PRINGLE, RUNNING BACK
A seven-time eastern All-Star, he made the Western All-Star team his first year in the division.

TERRY VAUGHN, SLOTBACK
His eighth straight selection to the Western All-Star team.

ED HERVEY, WIDE RECEIVER
His second Western All-Star selection.

DAN COMISKEY, OFFENSIVE GUARD
His first All-Star selection.

BRUCE BEATON, OFFENSIVE TACKLE
The seventh All-Star selection for this Eskimo ironman who hasn't missed a game since 1995.

Defense

DONNY BRADY, DEFENSIVE BACK
His first All-Star selection.

SHANNON GARRETT, DEFENSIVE BACK
His second All-Star selection.

Special Teams

SEAN FLEMING, PUNTER
The second All-Star selection for this 12-year veteran.

EDMONTON ESKIMO'S 2003 ALL-CANADIAN TEAM

MIKE PRINGLE, RUNNING BACK
His seventh All-Canadian selection.

ED HERVEY, WIDE RECEIVER
His first All-Canadian selection.

BRUCE BEATON, OFFENSIVE GUARD
His second All-Canadian selection.

DONNY BRADY, DEFENSIVE BACK
His first All-Canadian selection.

Contents

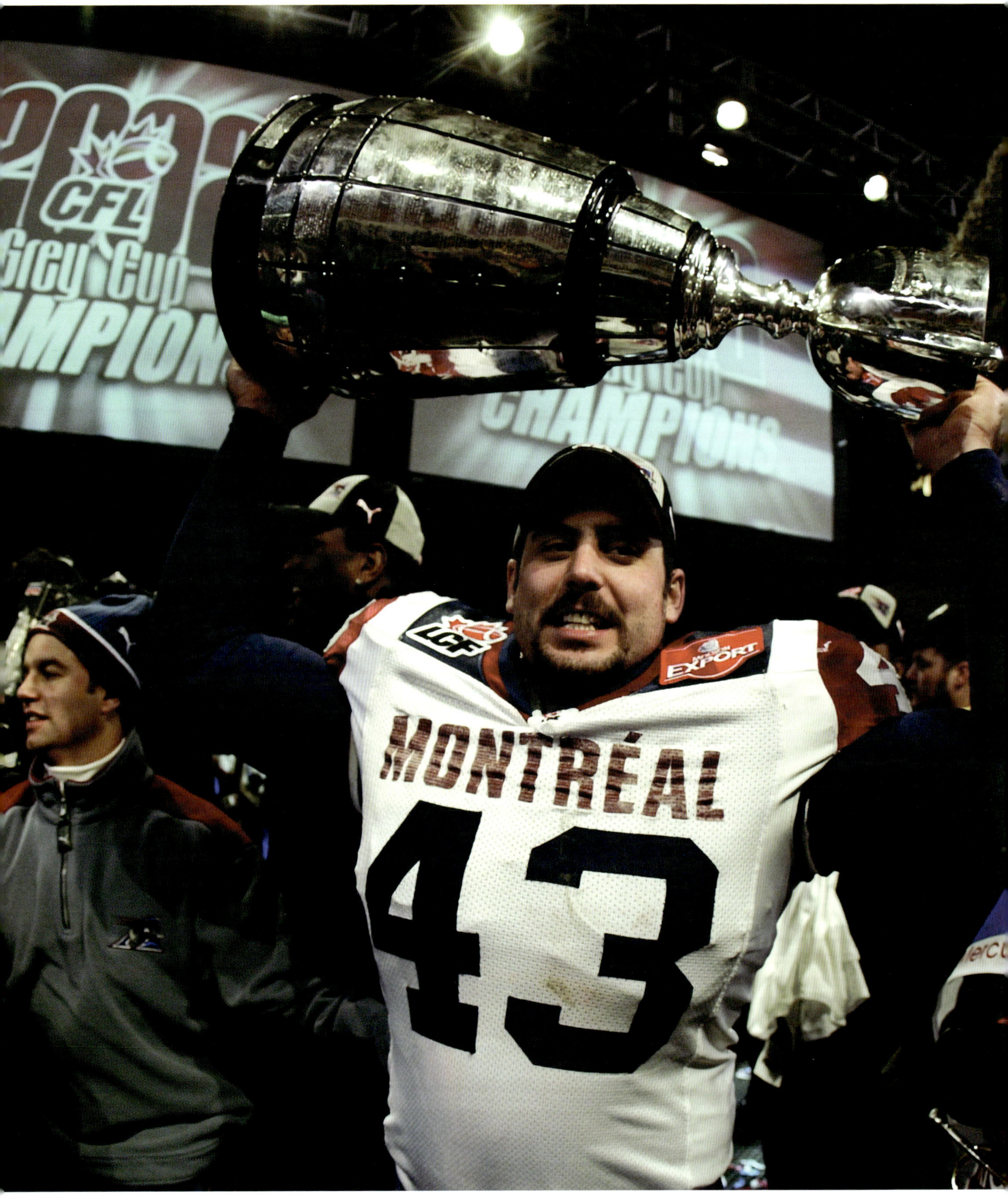
CFL
Grey Cup
CHAMPIONS
LCF
EXPORT
MONTRÉAL
43

Chapter 1

The Revenge of The Don

GREY CUP GAME 2002

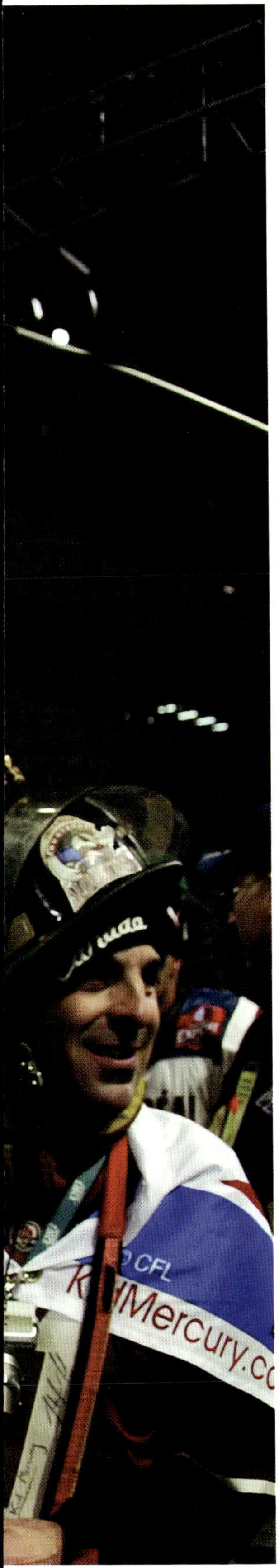

How sweet it is! Montreal tackle Jason Richards celebrates his first Grey Cup surrounded by supporters.

For the first time in the storied history of Canada's most distinguished football franchise, the Edmonton Eskimos would play for the Grey Cup at home. Commonwealth Stadium, November 24, 2002, would mark the ninth time the Edmonton Eskimos and Montreal Alouettes would meet for all the marbles. Before that, beginning in 1954, Parker, Bright and Kwong had run their way into the annals of Canadian sport by leading the Eskimos to three straight Grey Cup victories over the Montreal Alouettes.

The two teams would meet five more times in the 1970s, the Eskimos winning Lord Grey's cherished trophy on three of those occasions thanks to a new generation of green and gold heroes like George McGowan, Ron Estay, Dave Cutler, Tom Scott, Tom Wilkinson, Warren Moon, Brian Kelly, Dan Kepley and Dave Fennell. After their 1979 clash at Montreal's Olympic Stadium, won by the Eskimos 17–9, Edmonton would continue to add to their legacy of greatness by winning the Holy Grail of Canadian football five times in eight attempts. Future Hall of Famers Matt Dunigan and Damon Allen did the honors, followed by the dynamic duo of Danny McManus and Darren Flutie. In the meantime, the Alouettes folded just before the first regular season game in 1987. CFL football returned to Montreal nine years later when the defending Grey Cup champion

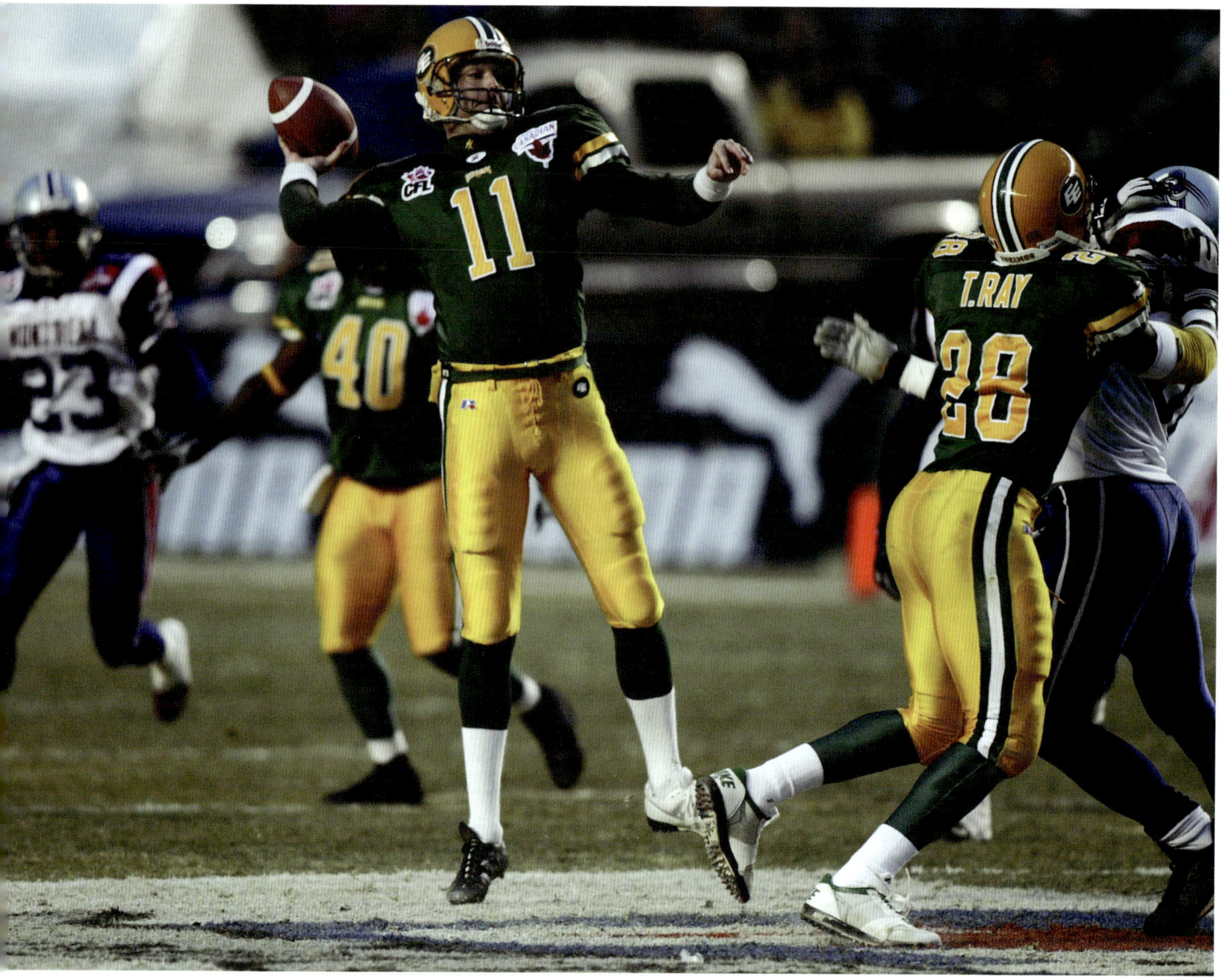

After his punt was blocked, Sean Fleming recovered the ball and threw to Donny Brady. It was incomplete, but Mark Washington was called for interference.

Baltimore Stallions moved north, Canadian Football League expansion to the United States a shattered dream. Six years later, the historic rivalry would be renewed.

Hard times had uncharacteristically fallen upon the Edmonton Eskimos. Although they had not missed the play-offs since 1971, they had gone nine years without a Grey Cup. Whether it be hiring National Cash Register salesman Norm Kimball to be minor football coordinator and general manager, or 32-year-old Ray Jauch as head coach, succeeded by Whitworth College mentor Hugh Campbell and later Jackie Parker, Joe Faragalli and Ron Lancaster, the Eskimos had always shown a genius for hiring exactly the right personnel.

But President Hugh Campbell made a disastrous mistake when he replaced his old pal Ronnie with Kay Stephenson in 1998. He soon corrected his error by turning back to the Eskimo family and convincing another old friend, Don Matthews, to leave the Good Ship Argonaut and return to the Igloo.

Perhaps you can't go home again. Rebuilding in 1999, Matthews experienced the only losing season of his head coaching career, finishing 6–12 in third place and bowing to Calgary in the semifinal 30–17. In the first season of the new millennium, he did slightly better, moving up to second place at 10–8. Again the Eskimos lost the semifinal, this time to B.C. 34–32.

During Matthews' third training camp in Edmonton, Campbell took the incredible step of firing his friend, ostensibly for missing practices and generally neglecting his duties. Matthews said he had a thyroid problem and had been forgetting to take his medication. He was angry and devastated. That December, President Larry Smith and another old friend, General Manager Jim Popp, hired him to coach the Alouettes.

After finishing first with a record of 13–5 and an Eastern final victory over Toronto, Matthews prepared to return to Edmonton for the 90th playing of the Grey Cup. To have said there was bad blood before the big game would have been an understatement. The most successful head coach in CFL history vowed revenge.

His replacement on the Esks' bench was the team's genial, bespectacled general manager, Tom Higgins. When he got the call from Campbell to replace a living legend, the only head coaching experience at any level the North Carolina State graduate had was of his son's bantam team, which he left to assume control of the Eskimos. Higgins worked hard to replace the popular Matthews and to secure the team's respect and loyalty. The team went 9–9, generally a mediocre mark in the ever-so-tough Western Division but good enough for first place and a bye to the Division final in 2001. They lost that game at home to the 8–10 Stampeders 38–16. Given the circumstances he faced, Higgins had done a great job to get that far. He didn't think so.

"We finished the season on what our players considered as low a note as you can. We didn't play as well as we would like to have played. If we had played better and lost, it might have been not as bad an off-season as it was, but to play as poorly as we did against Calgary in the Western final means we would like to have another opportunity at it."

He would get that opportunity six months later.

Higgins had every reason to be optimistic. He was so high on his All-Star quarterback Jason Maas that he traded backup Nealon Greene to Saskatchewan for running back Darren Davis and offensive lineman Dan Comiskey. When he talked about his quarterbacks before the preseason, he didn't even mention newcomer Ricky Ray. But when Maas was knocked from the game with a separated shoulder in the fourth quarter at

Taylor Field on July 19, it was Ray who stepped in and saved the day. He's been the starter ever since.

At 23, and the youngest starting quarterback in the league, how could this refugee from Sacramento State and the Arena League play so well?

"I always felt confident I could play. Obviously, I didn't know I was going to do as well as I did right from the start. You've got to make the most of your opportunities. You hope you can get off to a good start and get some confidence, and I've been able to do that.

"The strength of my game is being able to learn and pick up things quickly, make good decisions and just be relaxed and calm out there. In my first start against B.C. [a 37–27 win] I said to myself, 'Just play the game the way you've been playing; don't try to do too much. Don't try to impress everybody, just play your game.' I feel comfortable and confident that I can do all right."

Just before Ray signed with Edmonton on May 27, 2002, he was delivering potato chips for Frito Lay. His Fresno Frenzy Arena League coach, former CFL veteran quarterback Rick Worman, recommended his young charge to his old friend Tom Higgins.

"I played an arena game on Saturday night. My coach told me I had a chance to go to Edmonton right after the game. So Sunday I went back home, packed up my stuff and flew out Monday. From the time I knew I was coming to Edmonton and arrived here, it was only like 36–48 hours. It was just one of those decisions you've got to make, and hopefully it is the right one. When you come up here, you don't know anybody; you have a new country to adjust to; it's not easy but you stick it out."

Showing maturity beyond his years, Ray led the Eskimos to a 13–5 finish and first place. He was second in the CFL in passing, completing 227 of 359 attempts for 2,991 yards and 24 touchdowns. He had the highest passing efficiency in the league. He also had outstanding playmates to work with. The great Terry Vaughn caught 94 passes for 1,291 yards. Jason Tucker had 51 receptions and Ed Hervey 50. Chris Brazzell came on strong at the end. Sensational running back John Avery was the league's leading rusher with 1,448 yards and third in combined yards with 2,530. Elfrid Payton, the CFL's Outstanding Defensive Player of 2002, was No. 1 in sacks with 16, seven more than the runner-up, teammate Albert Reese.

This time the Eskimos did not falter in the Western final, beating the Blue Bombers 33–30. Ray completed 19 of 34 passes for 269 yards. Avery ran for 144 yards. Given the Grey Cup would be played in Edmonton, the Eskimo victory was extra special.

Montreal? Bring 'em on.

The Eskimos dominated the game statistically with a 25–7 edge in first downs. They had 126 yards more in total offense and a time of possession differential of 35:15 to 24:45.

But they shot themselves in the foot. Montreal didn't so much win the Grey Cup 25–16 as Edmonton gave it away with missed opportunities, blown coverages, dead-ball fouls, poor coaching decisions and dropped passes. True, Avery was held to six yards because of a hamstring injury, but the field was so slippery that in all likelihood he would have been ineffective anyway.

Montreal opened the scoring before a capacity crowd of 62,531 with a 68-yard Terry Baker single. At 1:58 of the second quarter, Anthony Calvillo hooked up with Pat Woodcock on a record-setting, electrifying 99-yard pass-and-run, making the score 8–0 for Les Alouettes.

"We tried to isolate him on one of the DBs who wasn't used to his kind of speed," Calvillo explained. "We happened to get them in zone coverage, got the ball to him and he just did the rest."

From then until the fourth quarter, the Eskimo defense held the Als to a field goal made just before the half. Montreal went to the dressing room leading 11–0. It could have been the other way around.

Early in the opening quarter, Montreal blocked a Sean Fleming punt. Fleming picked it up and threw an incomplete pass, but Lark DB Mark Washington was called for interference. Ray and Vaughn teamed up for a 65-yard touchdown that was called back when Chris Brazzell was called for holding.

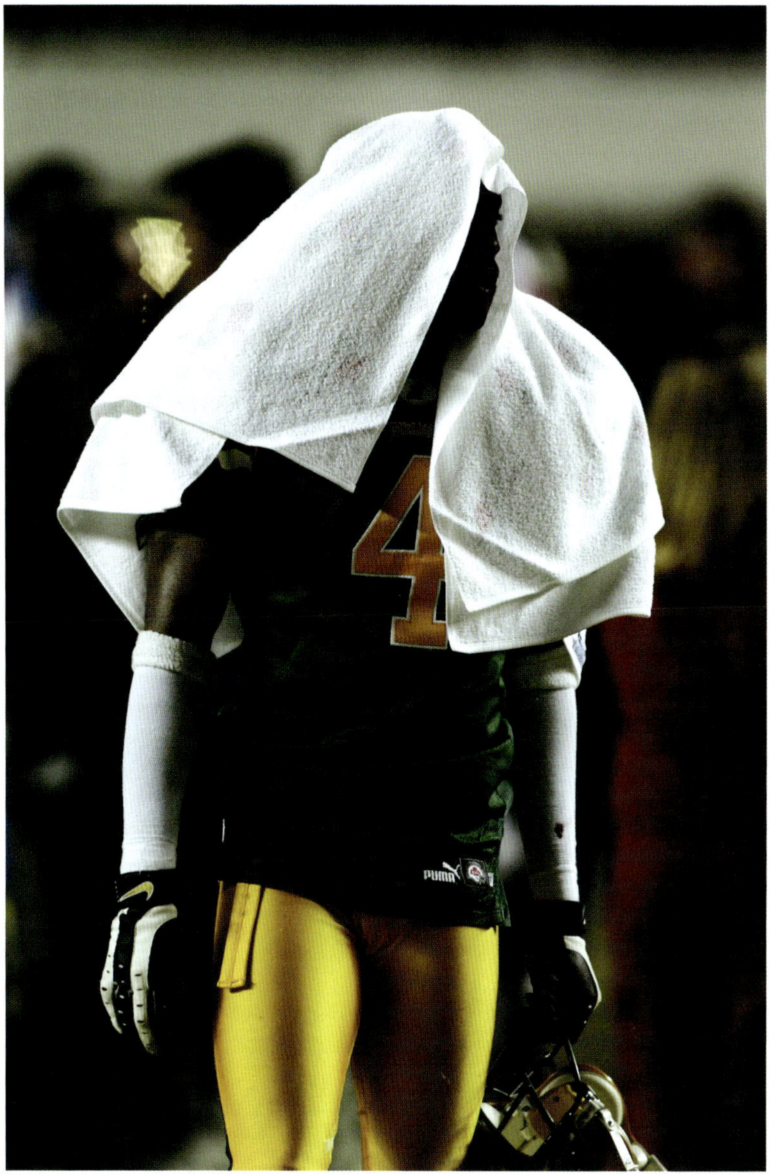

A despondent Darrel Crutchfield leaves the field.

Edmonton reciprocated the blocked punt in the second stanza against Montreal's Terry Baker, with Albert Kinney knocking the ball down and rookie Mike Bradley recovering. Although the Eskimos offense went two-and-out, the battle for field position had swung their way. Fleming's short punt pinned the Als on their 11-yard line, and one play later, Woodcock covered the 99 yards to the end zone. The Eskimos' next three possessions self-destructed when Vaughn missed a sure completion, Ricky Walters nullified a first down with offensive interference and Ray undid a march to the Alouette 20 by throwing an end-zone interception.

With the wind at his back in the third quarter, Ray completed a 38-yard strike to Jason Tucker. At the Alouette 18, he exploited a safety blitz and threw to Ricky Walters for a touchdown. Minutes later, after a Calvillo fumble, Edmonton closed the gap to one on a 13-yard field goal. Three turnovers, three points. Not good enough. In the last minute of the quarter, Ray missed a wide-open Brazzell and a sure six points.

Early in the final frame, Edmonton's Sheldon Benoit was called for roughing the passer, keeping an Als drive alive. On the very next play, Jermaine Copeland took a Calvillo pass 47 yards to the end zone, making the score 18–10. The crunch came shortly thereafter.

Backed up at his own 10-yard line, Calvillo threw two incompletions. Baker shanked the punt and Edmonton took over at the enemy 36. Vaughn was wide open for a major, but Ray underthrew it. Third down and Coach Higgins elected to gamble. Incomplete again. The Alouettes couldn't move the ball, but they took a couple of valuable minutes off the clock and punted the Eskimos back to their 16-yard line. Then Ray went to work, engineering a 15-play drive capped off with a 17-yard touchdown pass to Ed Hervey with 19 seconds remaining. With Tim Strickland all over Terry Vaughn, the two-point convert failed. When the Esks attempted the short kickoff, Jermaine Copeland returned it 47 yards to the end zone. Final score 25–16, even though Edmonton held the Als to a single first down in the second quarter, none in the third and just three in the fourth.

Don Matthews had his revenge. His team had played conservatively and avoided major errors. The Alouettes sat back and waited for the Eskimos to make mistakes and come to them. Then they pounced. The old cliché proved to be true: the team that makes the fewest mistakes wins. When the chips were down, the Eskimos were found wanting—and at home no less. Disappointment understandably prevailed in the Edmonton dressing room.

Afterwards, Ray said, "It's one of those games when you can think back and there are so many opportunities where it could have been different."

Higgins was philosophical. "Maybe before you can win, you have to lose. Today victory eluded us. Maybe that will give us a deeper resolve to keep us together and go back and get it next year. I hope this was the start to getting the Eskimos back into Grey Cups."

In his first year at the helm, Higgins got to the Western final. Year number two, his team went to the Grey Cup but lost. Now, 357 days later, in Regina, it was time to take step number three.

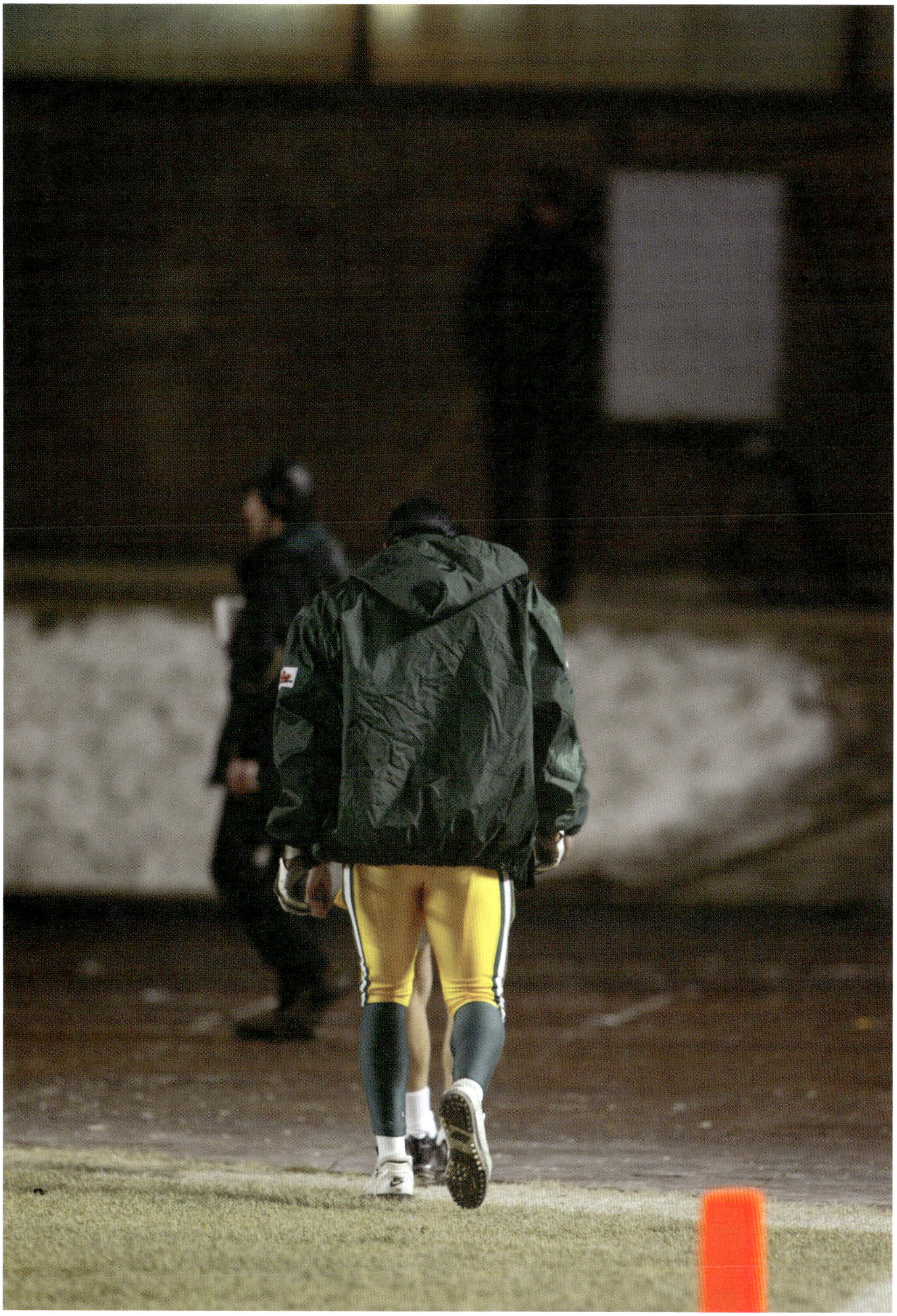

Running back sensation John Avery played his last game in green and gold in a losing cause. Later he signed with the NFL's Minnesota Vikings.

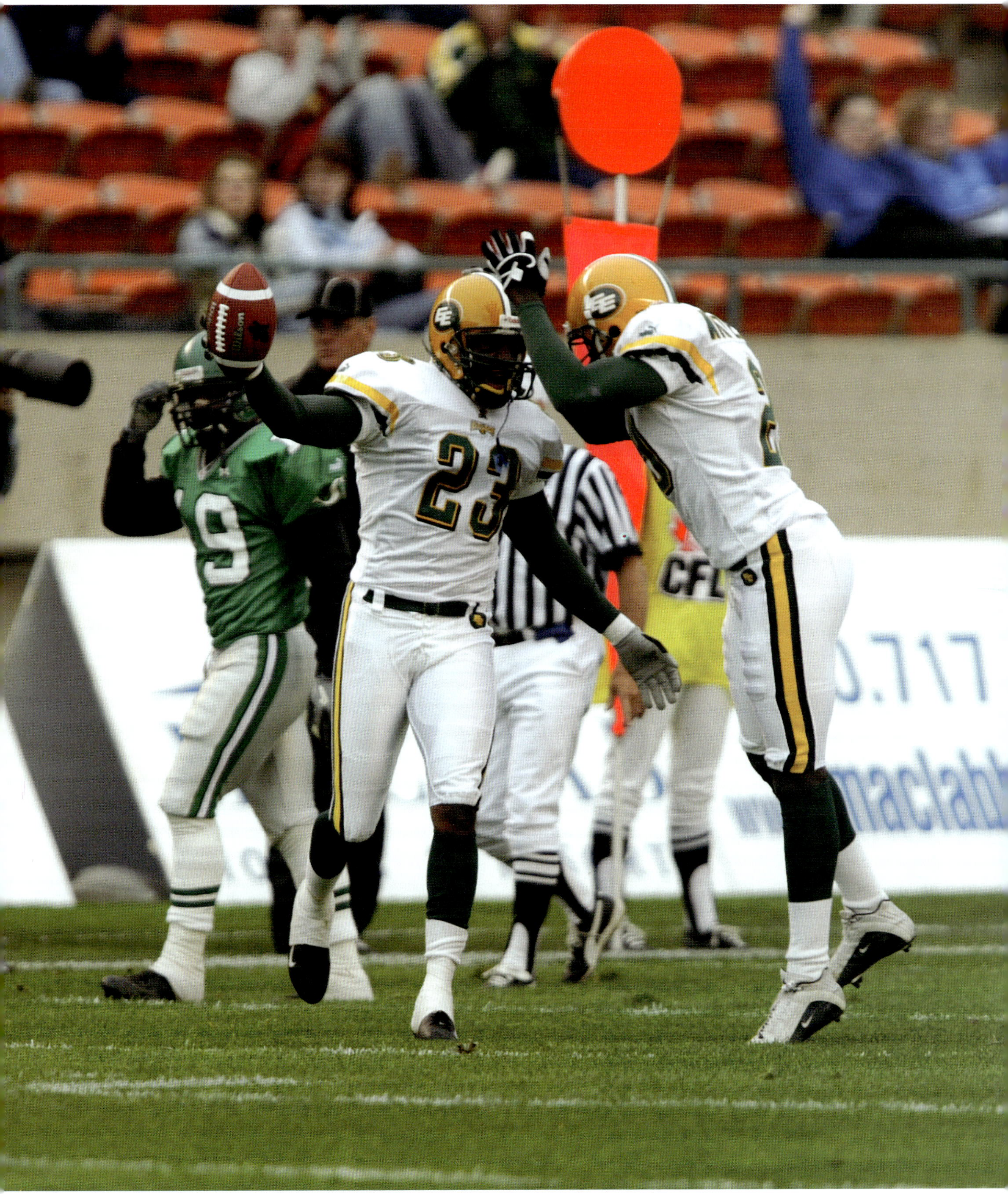
CFL

Chapter 2

The Best Laid Plans

PRESEASON & EARLY SEASON 2003

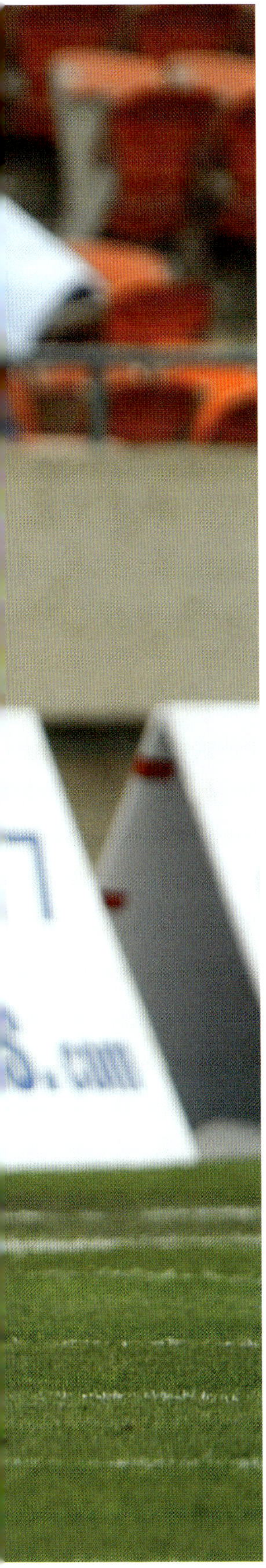

Shannon Garrett picks off a pass intended for Cory Holmes in pre-season action.

AFTER TAKING TIME OUT FOR THE HOLIDAYS, TOM HIGGINS and his staff began to prepare for the coming season, totally focused on returning to the big game November 16 in Regina. From 1999 on, the city that hosted the Grey Cup won it the following year. Whether it be talent or precedent, all the omens were favorable.

Even though his team had finished 13–5 and got to the Grey Cup, Higgins knew that to take the next step and bring the trophy home to the City of Champions, he couldn't stand pat. Age and injuries finally caught up to the outstanding homebrew defensive lineman Doug Petersen. The Simon Fraser grad retired after nine years in the CFL, four with the Eskimos. Joining him on rocking chair row was special teams star Jed Roberts, who spent his entire 13-year career in green and gold. The Grey Cup ring he won in 1993 when the Esks defeated the Blue Bombers 33–23 was the third for the Roberts family. His dad, Jay, earned two of them with Ottawa in 1968 and '69.

As Petersen's defensive linemate Steve Charbonneau observed, "It was a natural course of events. Everyone knew that Doug was going to retire. Physically, Doug was beat up. It was too bad for the game, too bad for the Eskimos because whatever he brought he was definitely positive about his attitude and the way he performed. Same with

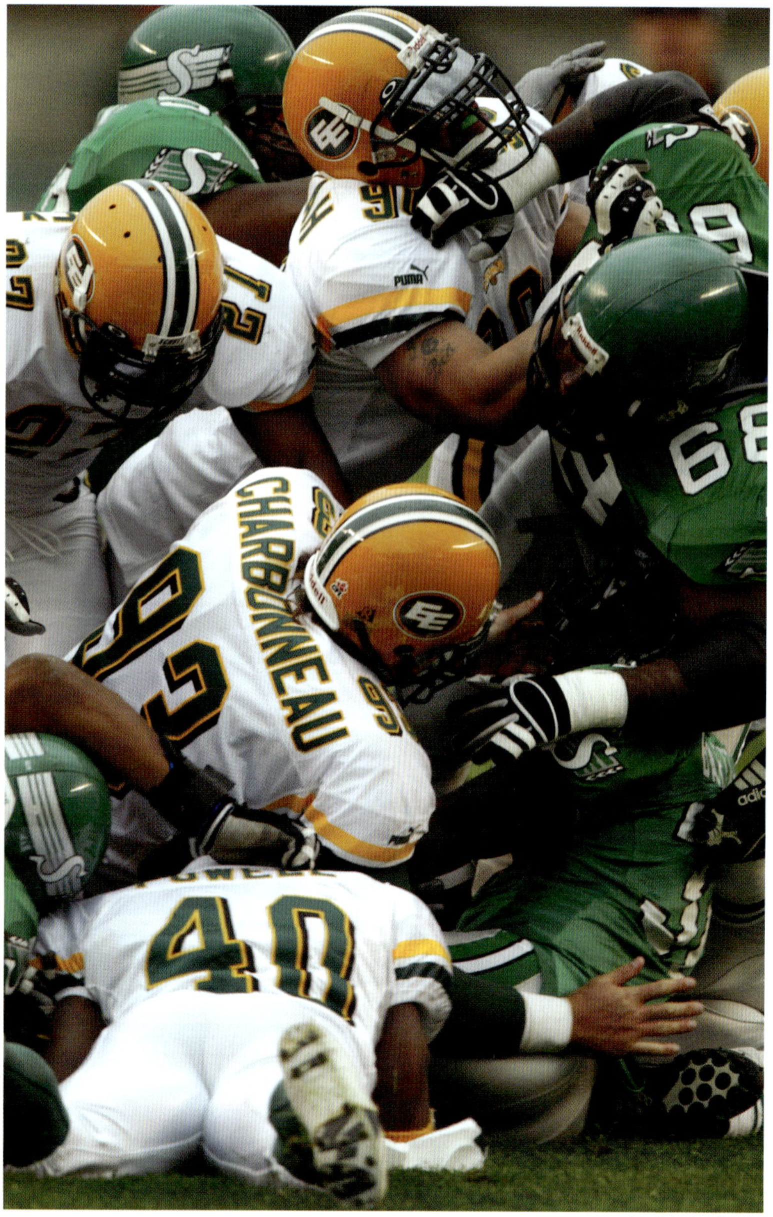

Trench warfare. Kelvin Powell, No. 40, Steve Charbonneau, Signor Mobley and Rahim Abdullah take on Saskatchewan's Andrew Greene, the CFL's Outstanding Offensive Lineman, 2003.

Jed. Their leaving left a big piece of the puzzle to figure out, but you've got to move on."

Others would move on as well, although not willingly. Determined to upgrade his secondary, Higgins released safeties Jackie Kellogg and Chris Hardy, eight- and six-year veterans respectively, as well as third-year man Jerome Peterson. Special teams star Justin Ring ended his eight-year career due to injuries, and Canadian linebacker Teddy Neptune was released. The talented but troubled running back Ron Williams was given his walking papers along with fullback Wendell Davis. Defensive end Kelvin Kinney opted for free agency and signed with Toronto.

The biggest off-season loss was running back John Avery, who led the league in rushing with 1,448 yards and was third in the CFL with 2,530 all-purpose yards. He took advantage of the CFL's agreement with the National Football League and signed with the Minnesota Vikings.

Higgins replenished his lineup with veterans. If imitation is the sincerest form of flattery, the coach showed his regard for the Alouettes by raiding their roster, signing Viking, Alberta, native Kevin Lefsrud to play right guard, and running backs Thomas Haskins and Mike Pringle. Former Eskimo Troy Mills returned to the fold after a year in Winnipeg.

Then things started to go wrong. The club announced on May 13 that Haskins would miss the season because of a benign brain tumor, having undergone surgery at St. Mary's Hospital in Richmond, Virginia, on March 26. Although the operation was successful, he couldn't continue his career. "First and foremost, I'm grateful to be alive, and I'll continue working towards regaining my health," he was quoted as saying. The all-purpose back would be missed.

Before the preseason, Coach Tom Higgins said, "We are making a conscientious effort to make sure our secondary and special teams are better. Some of the greatest battles in training camp are going to occur in the secondary."

Sixteen players vied to defend against the pass. No newcomers cracked the final lineup. To replace Jackie Kellogg and Chris Hardy, Higgins moved Quincy Coleman inside from the corner and replaced him with third-year man Darrel Crutchfield. Ageless veterans Malcolm Frank, Donny Brady and Shannon Garrett rounded out the defensive backfield. Predictably, they did about as well as the year before, but when the Grey Cup crunch came, they rose to the occasion.

In 2002, the defense gave up the second-fewest first downs in the league, but the team was fifth in points allowed. "We gave up a lot of points on special teams," Higgins explained. "Early on we were not very solid. The whole thought on playing defense is 'Bend but don't break, and don't make anything easy.' We had a lot of punts blocked that went for touchdowns. We had some returns on us. Points given up can be misleading. It wasn't the defense as much as special teams." In 2003, the Esks were second in overall points allowed (414 to Montreal's 409), but the Edmonton defense gave up the fewest points (367) and touchdowns (37). During the Labour Day Classic in Calgary, special teams breakdowns resulted in two returns of over 100 yards, both for touchdowns. But that was it for the season.

Winston October would lead the league in punt and kickoff returns with 1,018 yards and would be second to Toronto's Bashir Levingston in punt return yardage with 719. Waterloo graduate Mike Bradley returned the opening kickoff 92 yards to the house against Winnipeg on October 17. There is an old saying in football: "Offense sells tickets, defense wins football games, special teams win championships." What was a weakness became a strength.

The Eskimos of 2002 were plagued by fumbles and penalties. Higgins wanted to work on those areas, but, he cautioned, "It is an emphasis and sometimes the emphasis works against you. One of the things John Avery did beautifully was get yards, but he also put the ball on the ground a lot." However, it is still a team statistic.

"The discipline part starts from the very get-go—the hunger to make sure you don't take the avoidable penalties. There will always be some penalties, but many are avoidable. We have to make a concerted effort to do better." They didn't.

In 2002, the Esks had the most fumbles and fourth-highest penalty total. In 2003, they improved a notch in fumbles but were penalized more often and for more yardage. Untimely, turnovers and penalties would bedevil them throughout the regular season.

Higgins planned to start the

year with a defensive front four of Elfrid Payton, Rahim Abdullah, Steve Charbonneau and Albert Reese. But Payton, winner of 2002's Most Outstanding Defensive Player Award, injured his knee in the season opener and was lost for the season. There was some doubt whether Abdullah had fully recovered from a heart problem that felled him the year before. But NFLer Dorian Boose gave the team an outstanding fifth man on the line. The Washington State grad played three years with the New York Jets and 10 games with the Washington Redskins before signing and had been waived by the Houston Texans. Boose had seven sacks, and the Eskimos were second only to Montreal in total quarterback sacks.

Unlike Don Matthews who liked to send eight or nine players at the opposing quarterback, Tom Higgins got pressure from four. Although the spectacular Eskimo scoring machine would get most of the headlines, the defense was critical to victory.

And the defense, of course, includes the linebacking corps anchored by Terry Ray. Drafted by Atlanta in 1992, Ray played one season with the Falcons and four with the New England Patriots. After two years of failing to make NFL squads, he signed as a free agent with the Eskimos in 1999 and was a Western Division All-Star and Eskimo nominee for Most Outstanding Defensive Player three years in a row. A finalist for the honor in 2000, he lost out to Hamilton Tiger-Cats end Joe Montford. Ray made All-Canadian twice.

In a move that shocked and dismayed his teammates, Terry Ray was cut in favor of rookie Robert Grant, who joined the team right out of the University of Hawaii.

The story goes that Ray deliberately scheduled laser eye surgery near the end of May to avoid the detested rigors of training camp. Believing that Ray put himself above the team, Higgins let him go. It is more likely that Higgins believed Grant was so good that the rookie had to make the lineup and that Ray, 33, was in the twilight of his career. What ensued would tend to give credence to that claim. Ray signed shortly thereafter with Winnipeg but couldn't crack their starting lineup and had a miserable year. While some teammates like Singor Mobley roundly condemned the head coach for releasing the popular Ray, others took that and the injury to Elfrid Payton in stride.

Perhaps because of his generous nature, players have felt unafraid to criticize their head coach when he displeased them. Sometimes derisively referred to as Ned Flanders (Bart Simpson's Pollyanna-ish neighbor), Higgins is as smart a football man as you will find, coming by his talent honestly. His dad played in the NFL and coached football for 45 years.

Although the balding, bespectacled Higgins looks like a professor or chartered accountant, he was an All-American in football and wrestling at North Carolina State. He played for Calgary in 1976 and then shuffled off to Buffalo where he was a linebacker for the NFL's Bills for three years. After spending the 1980 season with Saskatchewan, Higgins retired to Calgary in 1981. He coached at Crescent Heights High School, then joined the coaching staff of the University of Calgary Dinosaurs, helping them win two conference championships and the 1983 Vanier Cup.

Higgins joined the Calgary Stampeders staff in 1985 as an assistant to Steve Buratto. For five years Higgins coached linebackers, defensive line, offensive line and special teams. In 1990, he became the assistant head coach.

When the Stampeders fired then head man Bob Vespaziani in 1987, the executive chose Lary Kuharich over Higgins as a replacement. Two years later, when Crazy Lary cleaned out his desk in the middle of the night and fled to Vancouver, Higgins was again overlooked in favor of his assistant coaching colleague Wally Buono. When it was clear Buono was settling in for a long run, Higgins joined the Eskimos as their assistant general manger in 1993, filling the vacancy left by Bruce Lemmerman's departure to the New Orleans Saints. In 1997, Higgins became the General Manager and Chief Operating Officer. Successful at everything he does, he has a .700 winning percentage, proving that nice guys can finish first.

But he replaced a legend. Many of the veterans Don Matthews brought to Edmonton attended his farewell press conference. Higgins said nothing. When Matthews criticized him to others, Higgins held his tongue. Positive and upbeat but understanding, he practices his Christianity by turning the other cheek. Because he is perceived in some quarters as a mild-mannered substitute for the real thing, when the Eskimos faltered, there were calls for his head and some grumbling in the dressing room. He took it all in stride. Charbonneau recognized the difficulties his coach and teammates faced in 2003.

"We overcame a lot of things," Charbonneau explained. "The Terry Ray situation was obviously a club decision. They had to make a huge decision to make room [for Robert Grant]. We knew that Ray had helped us the year before. The club had to make a decision, and they did. Elfrid getting hurt was too bad. With things like that you have to adjust from week to week, game to game. It is the same thing in life and the Eskimo organization."

Grant filled in admirably, making five interceptions, second best on the team. For part of the year he started because A.J. Gass was hurt. When Gass returned, sophomore Kelvin Powell was lost for the season. The only linebacking con-

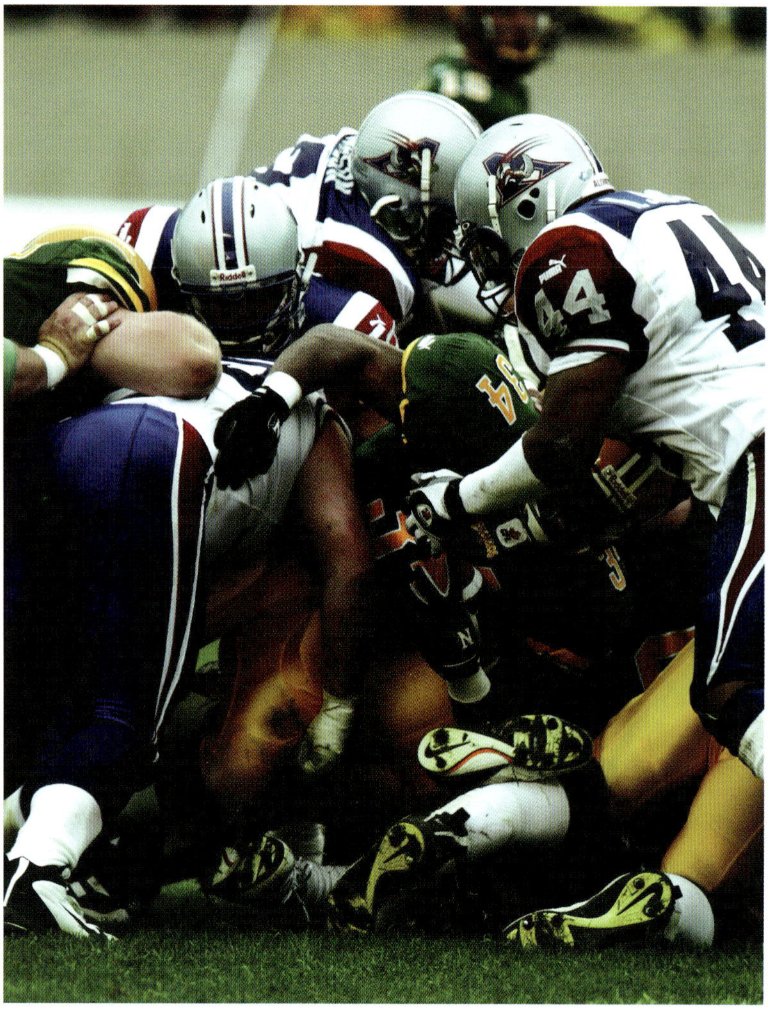

Mike Pringle attracts a crowd.

stants were the rookie Grant and the great veteran Mobley, who could always walk the talk—in his case an incredible feat.

Offensively, Higgins was convinced Mike Pringle could recover from a knee injury and a year of relative inactivity to be a game-breaker in the Edmonton backfield. Knowing Pringle's pride was hurt when he was relegated to the sidelines in favor of the flashier Lawrence Phillips, Higgins knew this great, proud athlete had a burning desire to prove Don Matthews wrong. Pringle would finish the 2003 season second to Winnipeg's Charles Roberts in rushing with 1,376 yards, the eighth time in the past 10 seasons that Pringle topped the century mark in rushing. If he faltered, another wily old veteran, Troy Mills, could carry the mail.

The receiving corps looked good in June with Terry Vaughn, Jason Tucker, Ed Hervey, Scott Robinson, Winston October and Ricky Walters. Pringle would catch 46 passes out of the backfield. The veteran offensive line of Bruce Beaton, Dan Comiskey, Tim Prinsen, Kevin Lefsrud, Chris Morris, rookie Carlo Panaro and Leo Groenewegen—who was entering his 17th season in the CFL—would certainly give the quarterback time to find them. But who would that quarterback be?

After graduating from Oregon in 1999, Jason Maas signed with the Baltimore Ravens but didn't make the cut. Coming to the Eskimos on March 21, 2000, he backed up Nealon Greene, seeing action only in the season opener. The following year he replaced Greene in Game 7 and never looked back. He was the West Division All-Star quarterback and Edmonton's nominee for Most Outstanding Player. In Week 2 of the 2002 season, Maas was named the CFL Player of the Week after completing 15 of 29 passes for 353 yards and two touchdowns against the Ottawa Renegades. On July 19 in Regina, he suffered a separated shoulder and, just as Nealon Greene had lost his starting job to the sensational Jason Maas, he in turn was supplanted by another young sensation, Ricky Ray. Maas later sustained a back injury.

Tom Higgins set improvement goals for his quarterbacks.

"Continued consistency," he explained. "The ability to grow. The only way two quarterbacks can grow is with experience, and we gained it for both Ricky Ray and Jason Maas. It was a tumultuous year [2002], more for Jason Maas because all of a sudden circumstances were such that Ricky Ray became a household name."

Although he was delighted to have two starting quarterbacks and potentially a third in Bart Hendricks, Higgins realized there was only one ball and all three wanted it. That concerned him.

"We have three quarterbacks who all want to play," he noted. "You need to address it; you need to discuss it early. They don't have to like it, but they just have to understand that it is the coach's prerogative and this is how the coach chooses to utilize his quarterbacks. I anticipate us as using a two-quarterback system. That is serving us very well. If we should have an injury, our season's not over because we have another quarterback who can step in and has been playing." He later would rethink his quarterback-by-committee plan.

After winning both preseason games, defeating Saskatchewan 17–10 and B.C. 38–9, the Edmonton Eskimos prepared to begin the 2003 regular season. Their goal from the moment Grey Cup 2002 ended was to get to Regina on November 16. Other than Kevin Lefsrud and Mike Pringle, only two newcomers cracked the starting lineup: Dorian Boose from the NFL and Robert Grant from the Aloha State.

They would open the season at home against Don Matthews and the defending champion Montreal Alouettes.

Although Cal Murphy was scouting for the Indianapolis Colts, his namesake's law prevailed in Game 1: If anything can go wrong, it will. Montreal continued their domina-

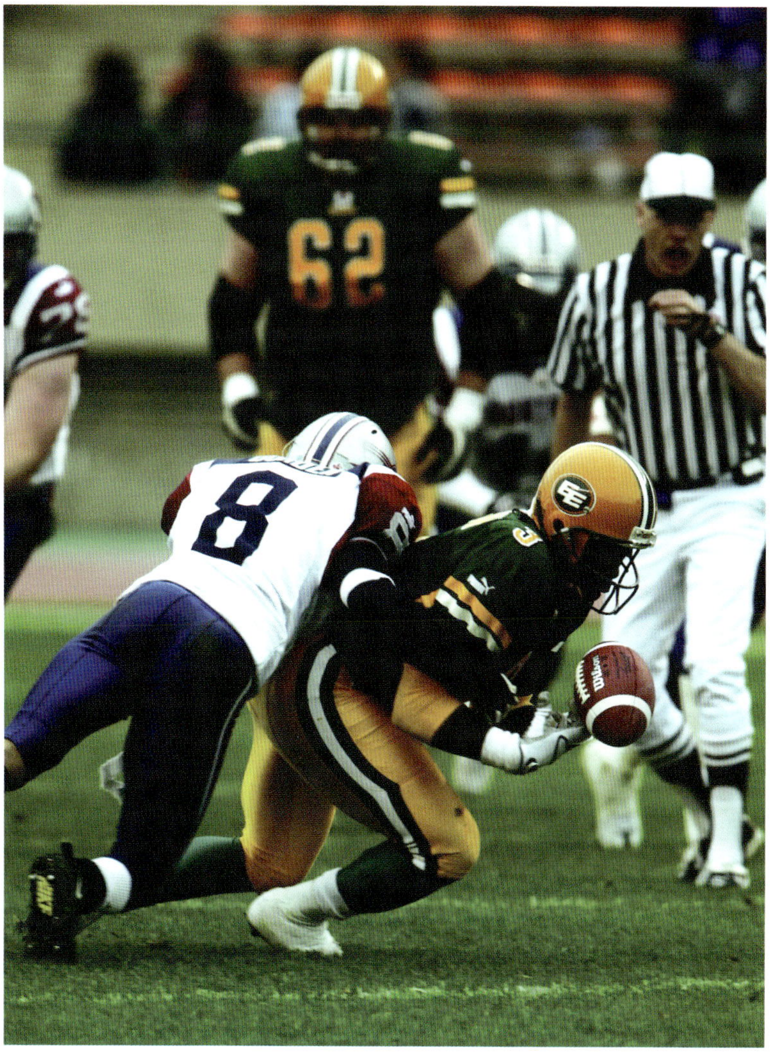

The season opener against Montreal was billed as a Grey Cup rematch. Alouette Reggie Durden prevents Terry Vaughn from catching a pass while No. 62 Bruce Beaton and No. 75 Ed Philion look on. Montreal won 34-16.

tion over Edmonton by winning 34–16, even though they were playing their second game in five days. While Higgins' goals included more disciplined play and better effort from the special teams and secondary, the Eskimos were penalized 22 times for 160 yards, gave up 214 yards on returns and 316 yards through the air, all of which nullified an excellent outing by the offense.

Ricky Ray was good on 22 of 31 passes for 241 yards and two touchdowns. Terry Vaughn had eight receptions for 118 yards and a major. Ricky Walters and Jason Tucker had eight catches for 88 yards while Winston October returned five kickoffs for 103 yards. Before leaving the field with an injury, Elfrid Payton rang up his 149th career sack, leaving him second all-time, eight behind Grover Covington. Still, once again, the Eskimos were their own worst enemy against the Alouettes.

Down Highway No. 2 to play the sad-sack Calgary Stampeders, the first of a three-game road trip, the Eskimos went. Calgary had been the dominant team of the 1990s under the direction of Wally Buono and Stan Schwartz, but new ownership had turned the franchise into a three-ring circus. During their home and league opener, the Stampeders battled the Alouettes into overtime. Trailing 23–20, new head coach Jim Barker opted to gamble on third down at the two-yard line rather than kick a tying field goal and allow the shootout to continue. It would be an exaggeration to say the Stamps never recovered, but that in fact is what happened. Calgary would finish 5–13, the opposite record of their hated rivals to the north.

Playing the second of what would be four games in 15 days, the Esks fell behind 18–3. Five minutes into the opening quarter, former Eskimo quarterback Marcus Crandell threw to former Edmonton receiver Don Blair for a four-yard touchdown set up by Wane McGarity's 79-yard return off Sean Fleming's 42-yard field-goal attempt. In the second stanza, Calgary's Mark McLoughlin kicked a 14-yard field goal at 2:23. Fleming replied 3 minutes and 47 seconds later. Crandell connected with newcomer Albert Connell for a 28-yard TD before Terry Vaughn dipsy-doodled through the Calgary secondary for a 17-yard touchdown just before the half. The score was 18–10.

Jason Tucker made an incredible flat-out, diving catch for a 27-yard touchdown early in the third quarter. Minutes later, Fleming propelled the Eskimos into a 20–18 lead with a 27-yard field goal. They won going away with touchdowns by Troy Mills and Tucker in the final frame. The Green and Gold had their first win of the season, 34–24.

Despite a slow start, Ricky Ray completed 21 of 31 passes for 331 yards and three touchdowns. Jason Tucker had eight catches for 171 yards and two touchdowns. Ed Her-

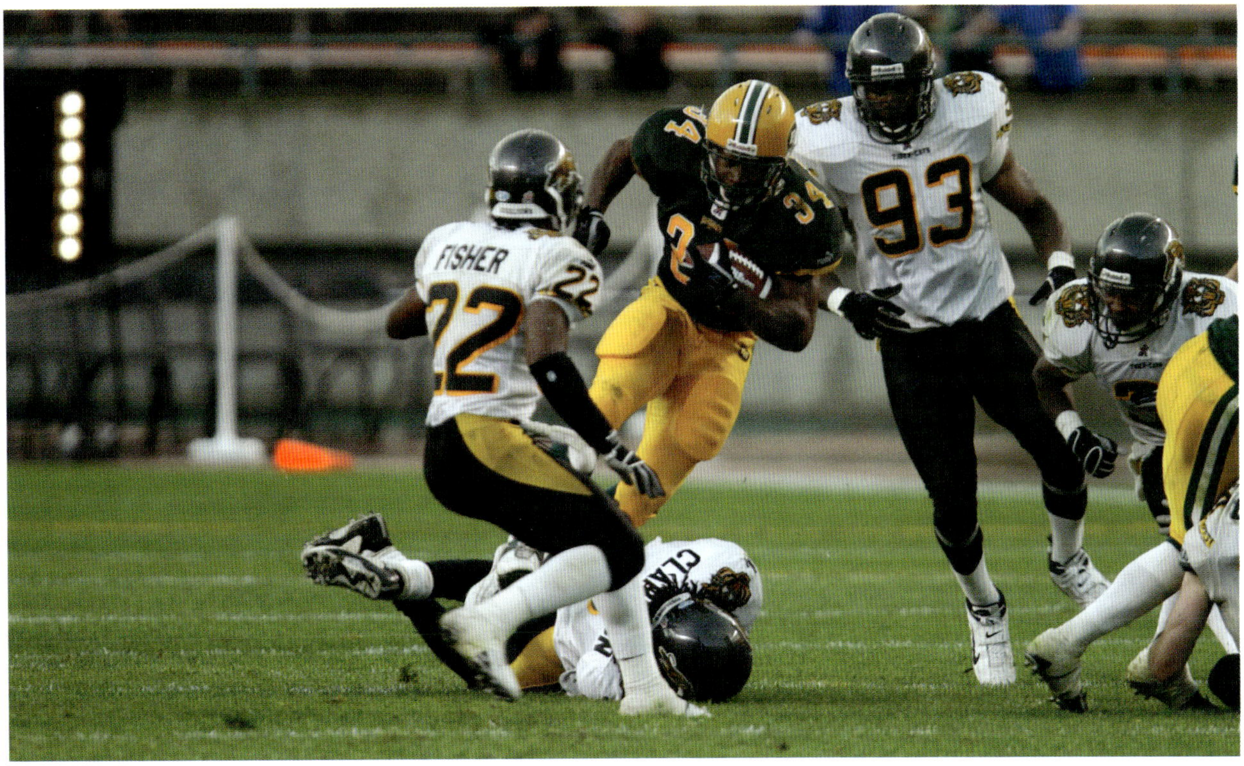

vey caught four for 99 yards while Terry Vaughn pulled in four for 30 yards and a TD. Newcomer Mike Pringle ran for 96 yards, becoming the second player in league history to crack the 14,000-yard career rushing mark. He would end the season 833 yards short of George Reed's career record of 16,116.

On to Manitoba.

When it comes to the Edmonton Eskimos, Winnipeg head coach Dave Ritchie and his Blue Bombers are in a perpetually grumpy mood. They've never liked Alberta in general, having lost the Grey Cup Game to the Stampeders in 2001 and the Western final to Edmonton the following year, all the while holding firm to their belief that they are the premier team in the CFL during the 21st century.

On Canada Day, Winnipeg got their revenge. Up against a ferocious wind at Canad Inns Stadium, the game turned into a kicking duel between Eskimos' Fleming and the Bombers' Westwood. Fleming was three for three in the field-goal department. Excellent special teams play by Roger Reinson forced a safety touch. Fleming added a 70-yard single. But 12 points were not enough. Westwood kicked two field goals, a single and a convert while Khari Jones hooked up with Milt Stegall, the CFL's Most Outstanding Player of 2002, for the game's only touchdown. A key play for the Eskimos came late in the game when Higgins opted to gamble on third down at the 24-yard line rather than go for what could have been a game-winning field goal. The final was Winnipeg 14, Edmonton 12.

On July 5, the Eskimos arrived

Mike Pringle on the prowl, Turrell Jurineak in hot pursuit.

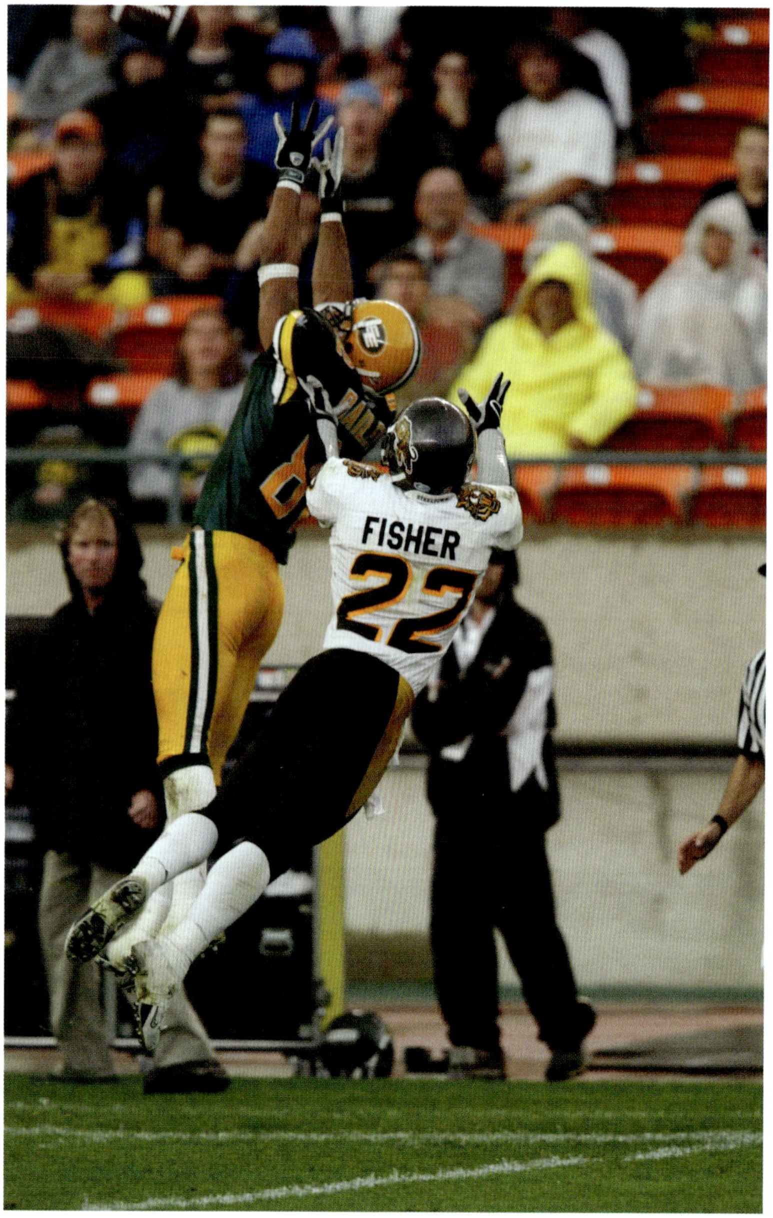

Kory Bailey out-jumps T-Cat Stephen Fisher.

in Steeltown, where one of the most disastrous seasons in Canadian football history was unfolding. Broke and soon in league receivership, Ti-Cat head coach Ron Lancaster couldn't make personnel changes because he was told by erstwhile team owners David Macdonald and George Grant there was no money to spend. He lost his veteran quarterback Danny McManus to injury during the season opener against Toronto. As former Roughrider General Manager Jim Spavital once observed about his own team, "If it costs a nickel to go around the world, we can't get out of sight." That pretty much summed up the predicament of a once storied franchise. They would win but a single game on September 12 over Saskatchewan. As McManus would say to a Roughrider player at the Grey Cup, "You guys prevented us from having a perfect season, 0–18."

Anxious to test his two-quarterback system, Higgins gave the ball to Bart Hendricks. The Boise State product engineered 10 quick points with a Pringle touchdown and a Fleming field goal. With second-stringer Pete Gonzalez at the controls, the Ti-Cats tied it up in the second quarter. Near the end of the half, Higgins pulled the now struggling Hendricks and went back to Ricky Ray, who combined with rookie Brock Ralph for his first professional touchdown. Rob Grant also tallied his first pro major when he returned an interception 71 yards to the end zone in the dying minutes of the game. Ray had another fine night, going 10 for 16, amassing 140 yards and two TDs through the air despite a sore left shoulder. Pringle picked up 125 yards rushing, tying George Reed's record of 66 career 100-yard games. Linebacker Kelvin Powell had a great game with five tackles, two sacks and a forced fumble. The Eskimos won 37–20 and returned home for a rematch against those same Tiger-Cats. Although it was only July 5, they had already played one-third of their away games and were undefeated on the road.

Typical of an organization with high expectations, they weren't satisfied with their play.

Back at Commonwealth Stadium July 16, Mike Pringle ran wild, picking up 149 yards to break Reed's 100-yard games record. He also scored two TDs. Ray completed 17 of 25 passes for 224 yards and four majors. Dorian Boose and Kelvin Powell each had three tackles and a sack while Ed Hervey and Terry Vaughn paced the offense with a combined 12 catches for 160 yards and three majors. Winston October was the special teams star with 92 yards on four kickoff returns.

On the opening kickoff, a Troy Davis fumble was recovered by A.J. Gass. Two plays later, Pringle scored from the five. Minutes later, Hamilton's Jason Currie missed a field goal, but Rahim Abdullah was thrown out of the game for dirty play. Hamilton kept the drive alive until rookie Julian Radlein plunged over from the one. Later in the first quarter, Currie conceded a safety touch, and October returned the kickoff 30 yards to set up Ricky Ray's 31-yard touchdown pass to Hervey. Leading 16–7 after fifteen minutes, the Eskimos poured it on. The final score was 52–15.

So what, the critics were saying. Beating up on the sad-sack Stampeders and two wins over hapless Hamilton were hardly signs of a dynasty in the making. Edmonton had lost to the only good teams they played, Montreal and Winnipeg. Next up in Regina were the surging Saskatchewan Roughriders. It wasn't a pretty sight.

Beset by a plethora of penalties in the early going, the Nealon Greene and White Riders jumped out to a 9–0 lead. Donny Brady got his team back into it by returning an interception 31 yards for his first CFL touchdown. Higgins replaced Ray with Hendricks, who failed to light a fire under the moribund offense. Meanwhile, Greene threw to Travis Moore for a touchdown. At the half, the home team led 16–8.

Higgins went back to Ray in the second half, but nothing worked. The penalties piled up, including an offside on a missed Paul McCallum field-goal attempt that soon resulted in a Chris Szarka touchdown run from the three. Fleming narrowed the gap to 23–14 with two three-pointers late in the quarter.

Higgins went back to Hendricks in the fourth, but Davin Bush picked him off for a touchdown to make the score 30–14. Fleming conceded a safety with 1:55 left on the clock. The final score was 32–14. A reflection of the intense rivalry between the two teams, four players were thrown out for fighting in the dying minutes, including Eskimos Bruce Beaton and Tim Prinsen. It would be the low point of Edmonton's season.

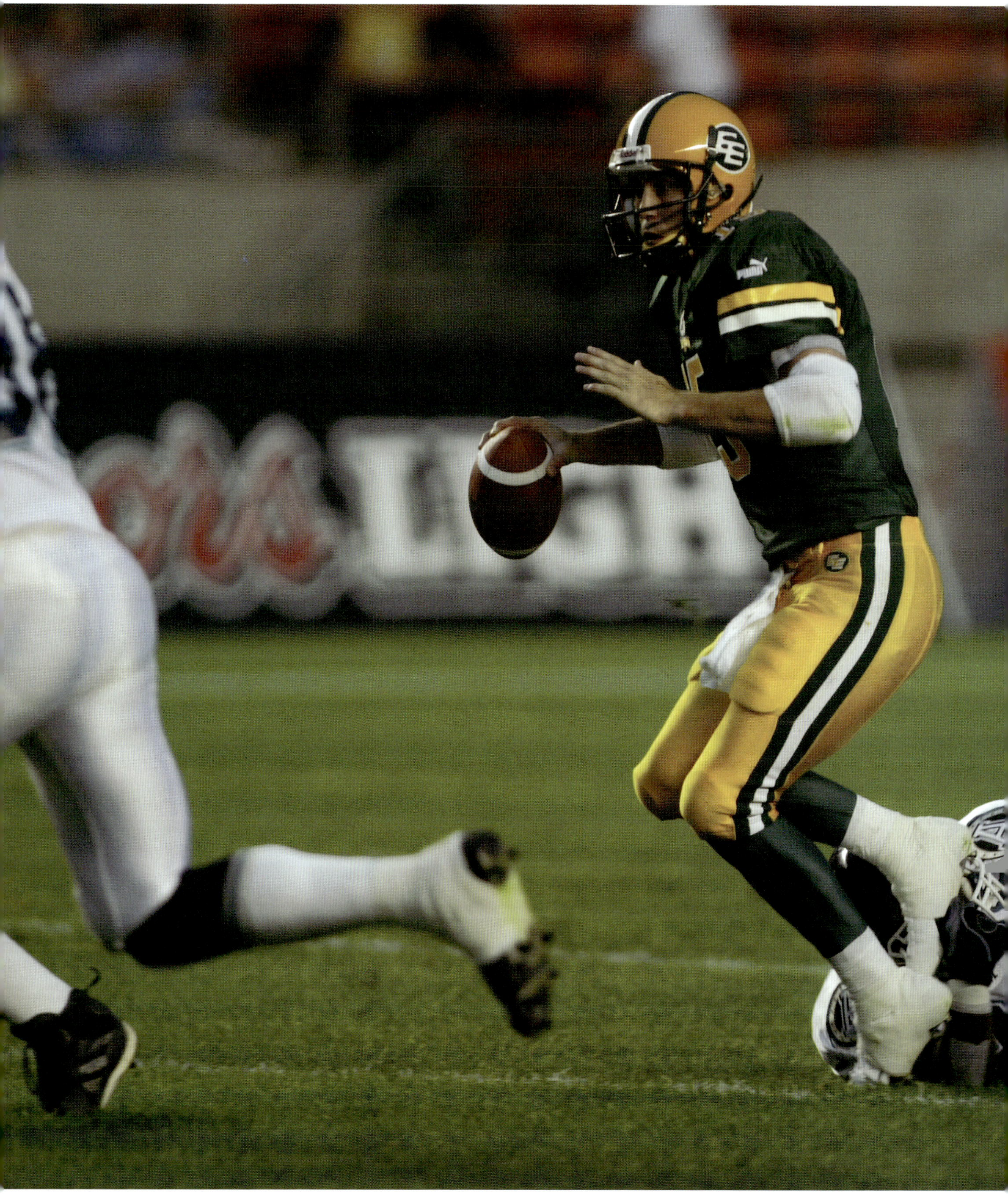

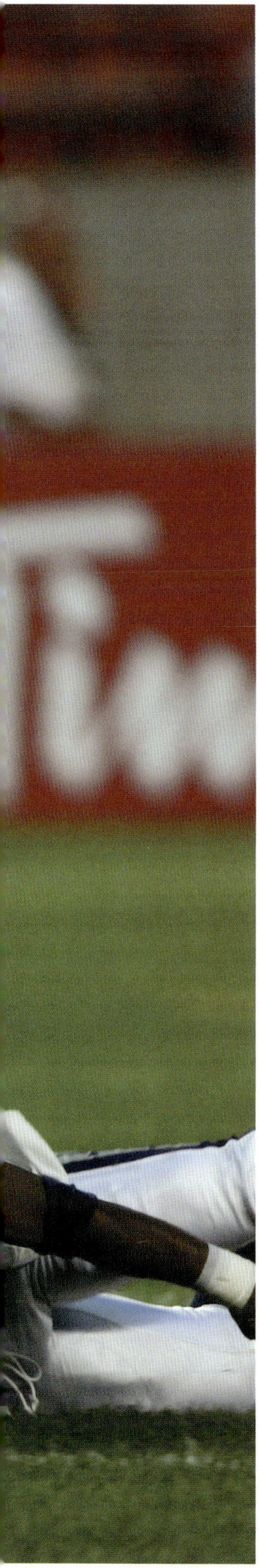

Ricky Ray sinks the Good Ship Argonaut.

Chapter 3

The Long Hot Summer

THE SEASON HEATS UP

A 3–3 RECORD A THIRD OF THE WAY THROUGH THE SEASON would be good enough for most of the teams in the CFL but not the Edmonton Eskimos. In all of North American professional sport only the New York Yankees and Montreal Canadiens have been more successful at winning championships. Only the Boston Bruins can match the 32 consecutive years the Eskimos have made the play-offs. Twenty-six Edmonton Eskimos are in the CFL Hall of Fame. Thirty-four Esks have won a league Outstanding Player Award, more by far than representatives from other teams. In their 55-year history, the team has made it to the Grey Cup 23 times (one more than the Winnipeg Blue Bombers), winning it on 12 occasions. But they hadn't won it for ten years and weren't happy with a mark of 3–3, which placed them fourth in the competitive Western Division.

On offense they were sixth over-all, with only Terry Vaughn ranked in the top ten receivers. Still, only the Lions' Dave Dickenson had a higher passing efficiency mark than Ricky Ray, and the bright light was Mike Pringle, whose 480 yards rushing was only two behind league leader Charles Roberts of Winnipeg.

Defensively, the Eskimos ranked fourth overall. Rookie Dorian Boose led the way with four sacks, followed by

Kelvin Powell with three. On his way to a berth on the All-Star team, Powell was fourth in the league in tackles. No Eskimo had more than a single interception. They were the most heavily penalized team in the league.

The good news was the Giveaway–Takeaway category, where their +5 mark was second only to Toronto's +11. Winston October led the league in kickoff return yardage. But 3–3 wasn't acceptable even though they were only two points out first place, shared by the Blue Bombers and the surprising Roughriders.

Steve Charbonneau was philosophical. "You win some, you lose some, right? I think every situation like the loss in Regina makes you stronger as a team. You go back and go to work. I think it happened for a reason.

"We knew that was not the club we wanted to be and we had to do something about it. We made a couple of changes on the roster, made a couple of changes on the defensive scheme and it paid off.

"I think it was just a matter of bringing everything together. The system and everything was good. It was just a matter of executing the system. There is no doubt in my mind that Greg Marshall has done a phenomenal job with the defense. We sort of got our stuff together.

"From day one of training camp, we knew we had the players to compete with anyone and be successful. The coaching staff had to make a lot of difficult decisions, and I guess they found the right combination."

It was off to the nation's capital for Game 7 and the beginning of a four-game winning streak.

The Ottawa Renegades were in their second year of existence, reborn six years after the demise of the Rough Riders. Randy Gillies, Kevin Kimsa, Brad Watters and Pat Paulin brought deep pockets, enthusiasm and expertise to the new franchise. They hired football genius Eric Tillman to run the operation. He brought in former CFL star Joe Paopao as his head coach. With a ragtag bunch of misfits and also-rans, the Renegades were 4–14 during their inaugural season. With former Eskimo quarterback Dan Crowley at the controls, they entered 2003 with a sense of optimism that wasn't misplaced. That wasn't because of Crowley—who was cut loose in July—but because of new quarterback Kerry Joseph and running back Josh Ranek. Legitimate stars like Kelly Wiltshire meant teams that took them for granted did so at their own risk. The Green and Gold almost learned that the hard way.

Ottawa jumped into an early 6–0 lead on the strength of two Lawrence Tynes field goals. They increased their lead to 13 when Joseph and Ranek finished off an 11-play, 96-yard drive with an eight-yard touchdown pass. The 21,200 fans in attendance at Frank Clair

Stadium could smell an upset. Ricky Ray promptly replied with an 11-play drive of his own that covered 69 yards. Jason Tucker scored the TD. Ottawa led 13–7.

Committing a rare turnover in the third quarter, Winston October fumbled a Pat Fleming punt that Denis Montana recovered on the Edmonton nine. The defense held the Renegades to three points. Again Ricky Ray answered the bell by connecting on four straight passes, bringing the offense to the Ottawa two-yard line, from where Mike Pringle battled his way into the end zone. The score was 16–14 for the surprising Renegades.

The two teams combined for 30 points in the fourth quarter. Jason Tucker scored his second touchdown of the night on a 21-yard pass from Ray, giving the visitors their first lead of the football game. Two minutes later Ray tossed a six-yard TD pass to Pringle. Fleming closed out the Eskimo scoring with a 28-yard field goal. Tynes added a field goal for Ottawa and Kerry Joseph threw to D.J. Flick for a touchdown. The final score was Edmonton 31, Ottawa 26.

Despite struggling through the first half, Ray was pleased with his performance, not because he completed 19 of 30 for 252 yards and three touchdowns but because he overcame a slow start. "This is huge for me to be able to battle through that and know that everybody has confidence in me. To pick it up in the second half is huge for my confidence and huge for me as a player."

The following week the Eskimos were home for the first in a back-to-back series with the Argonauts. Seldom a powerhouse, the Boatmen usually gave the Eskimos all they could handle, winning five straight at Commonwealth Stadium between 1996 and 2000. From '96 through 2002, Edmonton was 4–3 against the Argos at SkyDome.

With the Argos featuring former Eskimo great Damon Allen at the helm and an identical 4–3 record to the host, 44,205 fans came to celebrate Commonwealth Stadium's 25th birthday. They expected a close contest. It was anything but. What they got instead was a spectacular performance from Ricky Ray, who completed his first 14 passes en route to a 20-for-23 evening, 292 yards and two majors, proving he belonged in the pantheon of great Eskimo quarterbacks such as Jackie Parker, Don Getty, Bruce Lemmerman, Tom Wilkinson, Warren Moon, Matt Dunigan, Damon Allen and Danny McManus.

His favorite target was Terry Vaughn, who caught eight passes for 171 yards and a TD. Mike Pringle picked up 97 yards on 20 carries. The offense had possession of the pigskin for an awesome 39 minutes and 22 seconds.

Although the score was one-sided, there was no shortage of excitement. Return man Bashir Levingston ran a kickoff 95 yards for an Argo touchdown in the sec-

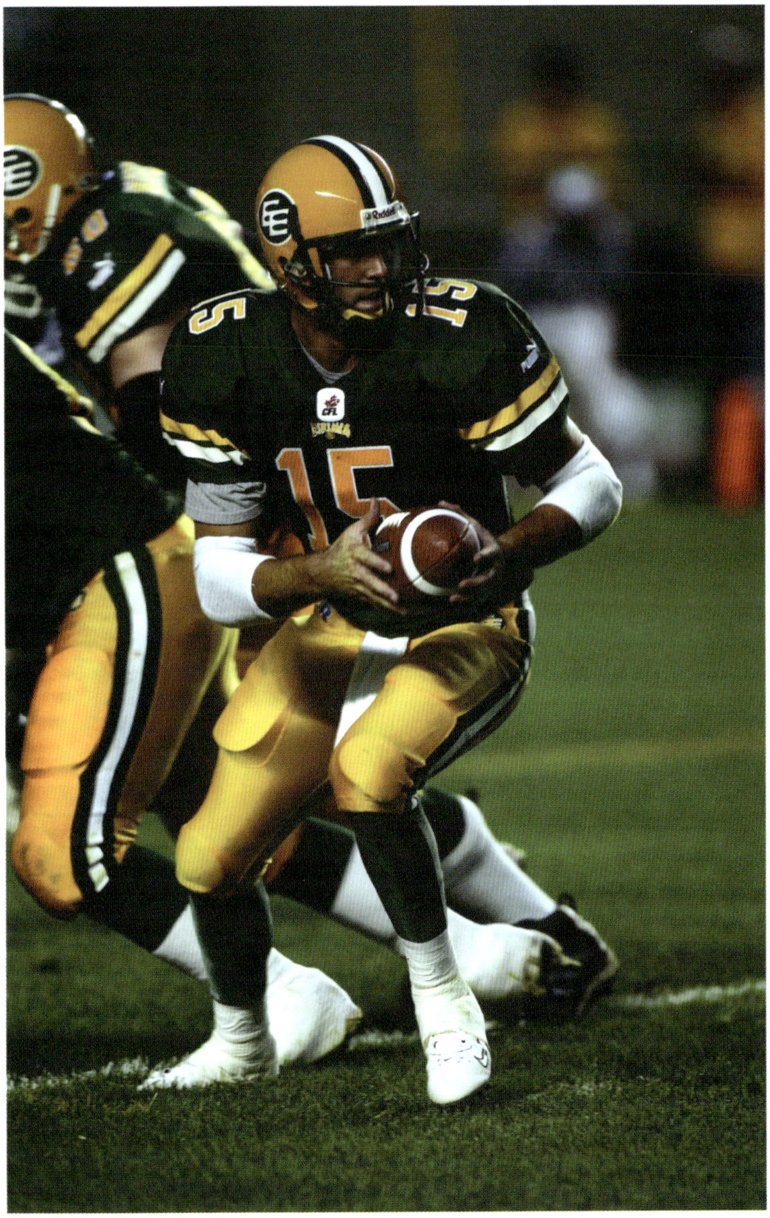

Where are you, Mike? Ricky Ray looks for a receiver.

ond quarter. Ray and Terry Vaughn combined for a 72-yard gain that would have resulted in a touchdown had Vaughn not collided with teammate Ed Hervey. Halfway through the third quarter, Ray strained a hamstring and was replaced by Bart Hendricks, who engineered two Sean Fleming field goals. Jason Maas came on as the closer and ran 15 yards to the end zone at 12:21 of the fourth quarter. The Eskimos improved to 5–3 by whipping the Easterners 49–20.

Back to Hogtown and the most bizarre experience of the Eskimo players' young lives. Scheduled to play Thursday, August 14, the game had to be postponed when a malfunction at an Ohio electrical station caused a massive power failure throughout the northeastern United States and southern Ontario. Already trying to cope with the SARS outbreak, which was devastating tourism, Torontonians were particularly hard hit. The least of their worries was Argo owner Sherwood Schwarz leaving the franchise on the CFL's doorstep and walking away. He'd lost millions and family members questioned his mental state for continuing to waste money on a football team that hardly anybody in Toronto cared about.

For the Eskimos, the layover in Toronto was a real life, if somewhat boring, adventure. They had to wait until Sunday to play the game. Naturally, most of them didn't bring enough clothes along, so shopping trips were mandatory. They expanded their horizons as restoration of power slowly spread throughout the region.

The first quarter was a study in ineptitude. Marcus Brady replaced the injured Damon Allen. Noel Prefontaine had apparently opened the scoring for Toronto by kicking a 40-yard field goal. But when the Esks were called for too many men, Argo Head Coach Pinball Clemons

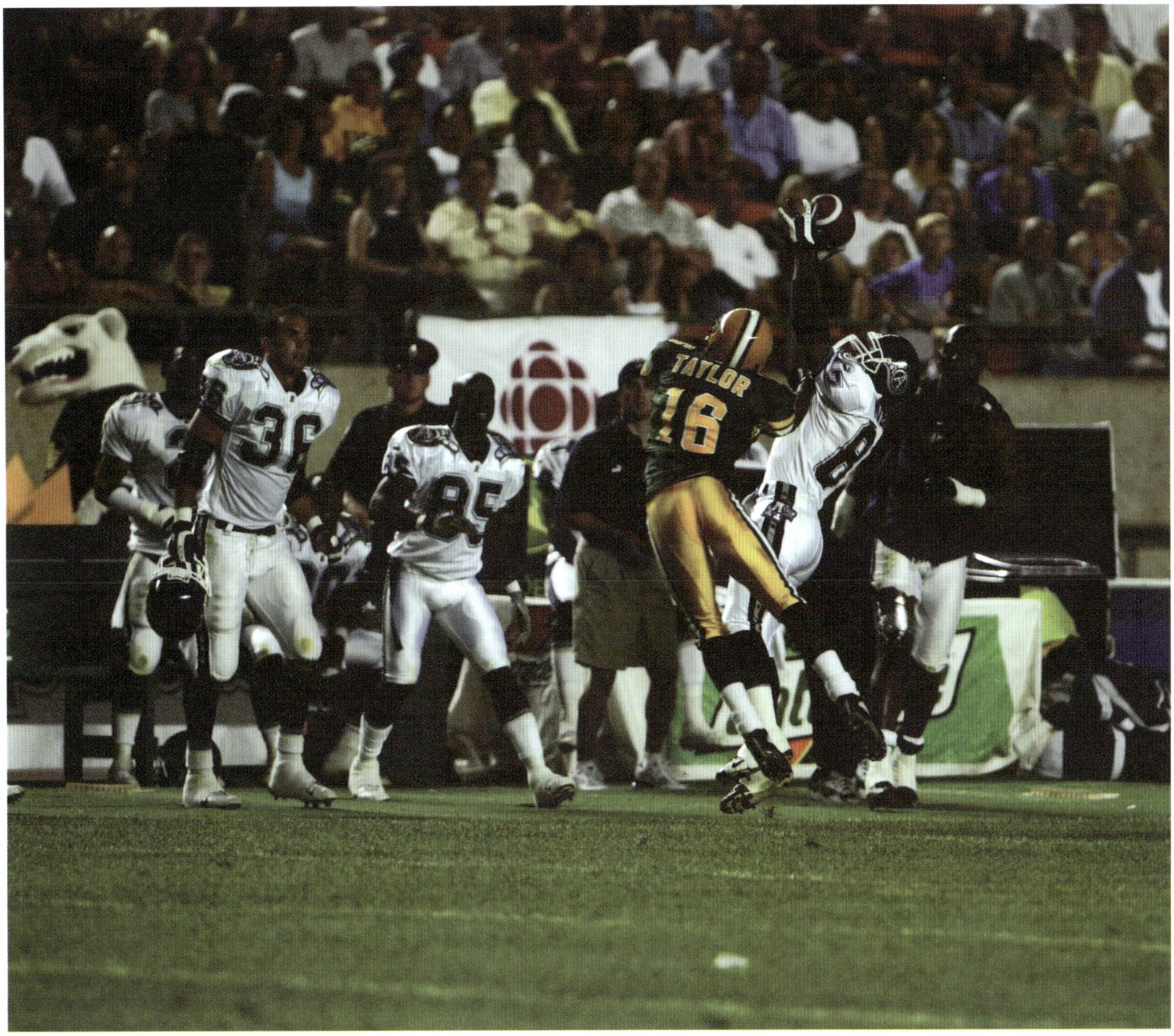

Cordell Taylor battles for the ball.

opted to decline the three points and line up at the 28 with a first down. After stalling at the 17, Prefontaine tried a 24-yarder that went wide for a single point. Brady was able to move the Argos at will between the 25-yard lines, but when they entered the red zone, the Eskimo defense stiffened and held them to a brace of field goals. After 15 minutes, the Argos were up 7–0.

The only scoring in the second quarter came on an Argo single six minutes in and a Fleming field goal with no time left on the clock.

The second half featured football follies at their finest. Fleming narrowed the gap to four points with a 14-yard field goal. On Edmonton's next possession, Ray threw 54 yards to Jason Tucker, who made a fine catch but fumbled the ball on his way to pay dirt. Tucker scampered back from the end zone to pounce on the errant pigskin at the Argo six. Two plays later, Troy Mills carried the ball the last yard into the end zone.

Prefontaine scored two three-

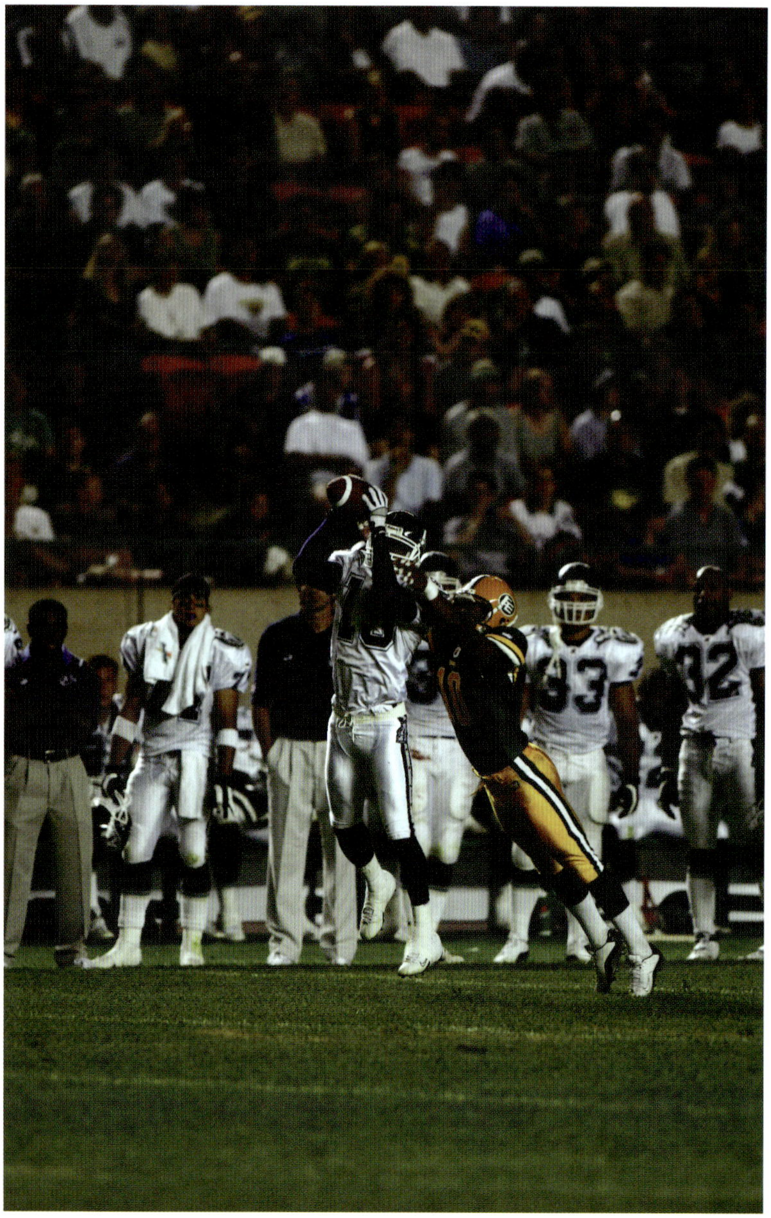

The always reliable Malcolm Frank shows how it's done.

pointers early in the fourth quarter to put his team ahead 14–11. Fleming tied it. After the teams exchanged singles, Ray drove his team into field-goal range with four straight completions. With one second left, Fleming kicked a field goal from 41 yards out, giving the Eskimos an 18–15 win. Afterwards, he gave credit where credit was due. "This was a game where we were definitely outplayed," he told the assembled scribes. "Our defense held us in and we're fortunate to have been able to get that last score."

Pretty it wasn't. Two points in the standings it was.

Over 45,000 fans welcomed the Eskimos home on August 23 for their critical contest with the Saskatchewan Roughriders. Because they had lost in Regina by 18 points, the Eskimos needed to win by one more than that in order to take the season series and the upper hand if a tie-breaking formula had to be used to decide play-off positions.

Going into the game, B.C., Edmonton, Winnipeg and Saskatchewan were tied for first with identical records of 6–3, Calgary bringing up the rear with two wins in nine starts. Because they had manhandled the Eskimos in Regina, the Riders came into Commonwealth with an arrogance and swagger that belied the fact they hadn't been playing very well. It provided a study in contrast of the two organizations. The Eskimos were 6–3 and believed they had to get better. The Roughies were 6–3 and smug. Terry Vaughn dismissed the Roughriders by calling them the Grey Cup champions of August.

After a couple of mediocre performances, Ricky Ray was on fire again. Knowing his team had to win by at least 18 points, he went right to work stretching the defense by going deep. But the opening

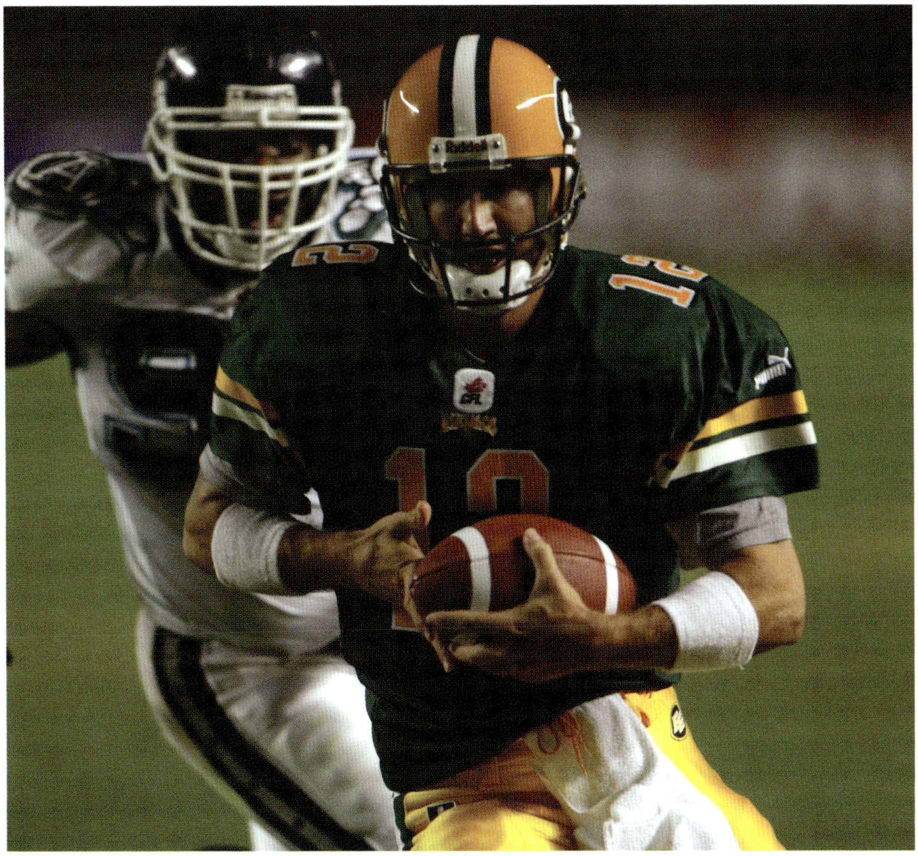

Jason Maas picks up a first down.

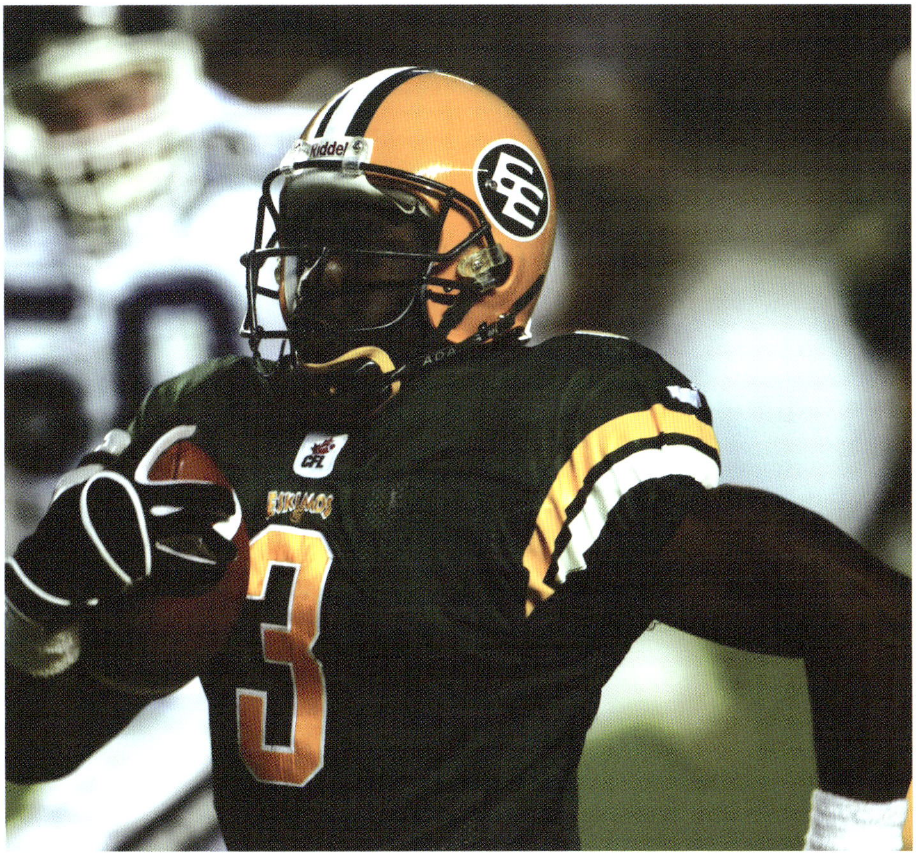

Terry Vaughn plays catch me if you can.

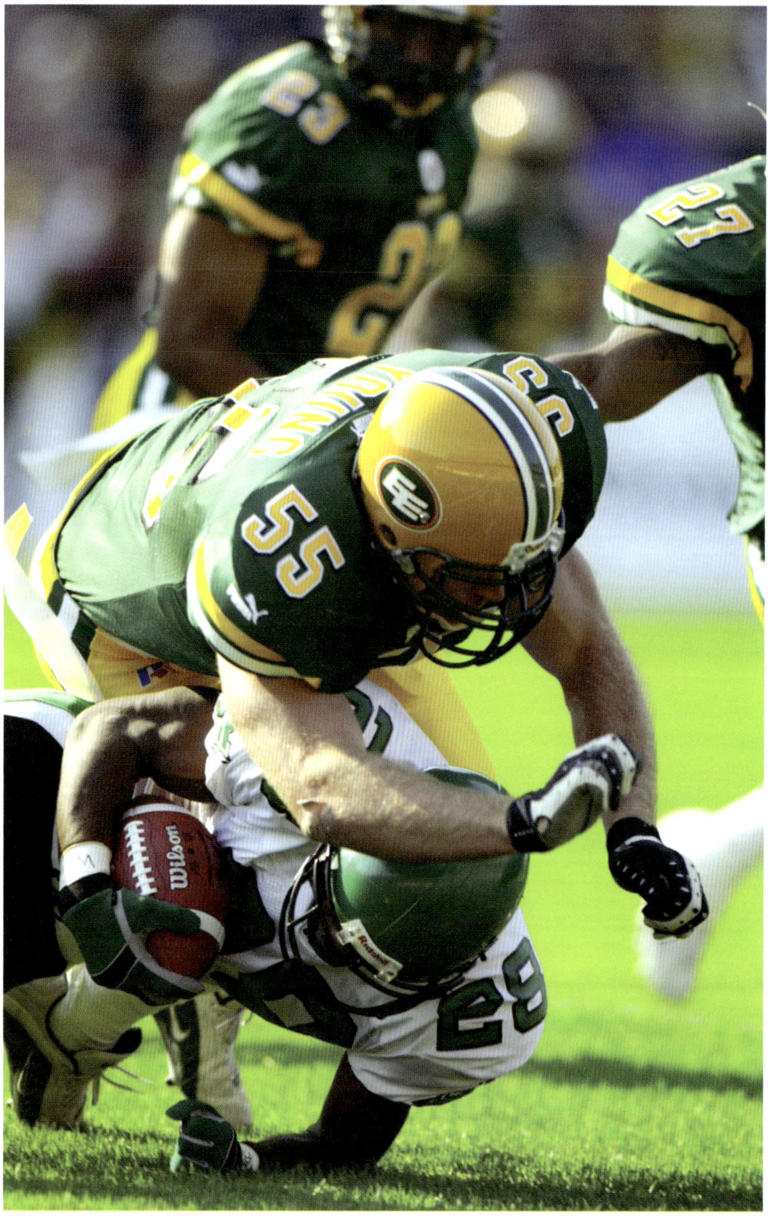

Linebacker Glen Young levels Kenton Keith.

drive stalled at the Rider 30-yard line. Sean Fleming missed the field goal try and had to settle for a single. On his next possession, Ray drove into enemy territory again. This time Fleming kicked it through the uprights from 42 yards out. On his third drive of the quarter, moving 68 yards in six plays, Ray threw to Scott Robinson for a 13-yard touchdown and a 13–0 lead.

Early in the second stanza, Rob Grant intercepted Nealon Greene and ran it back 45 yards to the Rider 24. Mike Pringle took it the rest of the way. Winston October set up a Ray-to-Tucker touchdown with a 39-yard punt return. That drive went 51 yards in six plays. Edmonton led 25–3 at the half.

The Riders began a comeback when Fleming fumbled the snap on a third-down punt at his five-yard line. Greene threw to Kenton Keith in the end zone. Ricky Ray responded immediately with a nine-play drive capped off with a 10-yard touchdown pass to Vaughn, restoring the Eskimos' 22-point lead. But on the final play of the third quarter, Corey Grant cut the lead to 15 points.

Pringle made it 39–17 at 3:24 of the fourth quarter. After the ensuing kickoff, Rider slotback Corey Holmes fumbled at his 35, recovered by Singor Mobley of the Esks. Two plays later, Pringle scored again, this time on a swing pass from 12 yards out. Edmonton 46, Saskatchewan 17—a seemingly insurmountable 29-point lead and an 11-point advantage in the season series. But remember, this is the CFL.

With a first down at the Saskatchewan 52, Ricky Ray ran to the 26, where he coughed up the football. Greene took advantage of the miscue and finished off a 12-play, 84-yard drive by running six yards to the end zone with 1:49 left in regulation time. Then Riders cornerback Omarr Morgan recovered a Pringle fumble at the Eskimo 50. Greene threw to Kenton Keith for nine yards; 15 more were tacked on for a face-mask penalty. That infraction was followed by two pass interference calls, bringing the ball to the one. Chris Szarka took it in with 31 seconds left on the clock. Edmonton's lead had shrunk to 15 points. Victory was secure, but suddenly Saskatchewan had a 63–60 advantage in the head-to-head points tiebreaker.

Riders defensive back Bobby Perry grabbed Winston October's face mask on the ensuing kickoff return, giving the Eskimos first down on their own 52. Ray got off three plays: a 14-yard completion to Vaughn, an incomplete pass rendered moot by the Eskimos going offside, and a nine-yard pass to Ed Hervey. On the last play of the game, Fleming kicked a 47-yard field goal, making the final score 49–31 and tying the season series at one victory and 63 points apiece. If the two teams were tied at the end of the regular season, points for and against each other could not be used to determine who would get the advantage.

Pringle had a great game, picking up 126 yards on 17 carries and 57 yards on five receptions and a touchdown. Ricky Ray from Frito Lay completed 24 of 33 for 311 yards, four majors, no interceptions. Vaughn walked the talk with five catches for 90 yards and a touchdown.

That same weekend, the Lions defeated Hamilton 47–25, and Winnipeg thumped Calgary 52–17. There was now a three-way tie for first among the Lions, Blue Bombers and Eskimos.

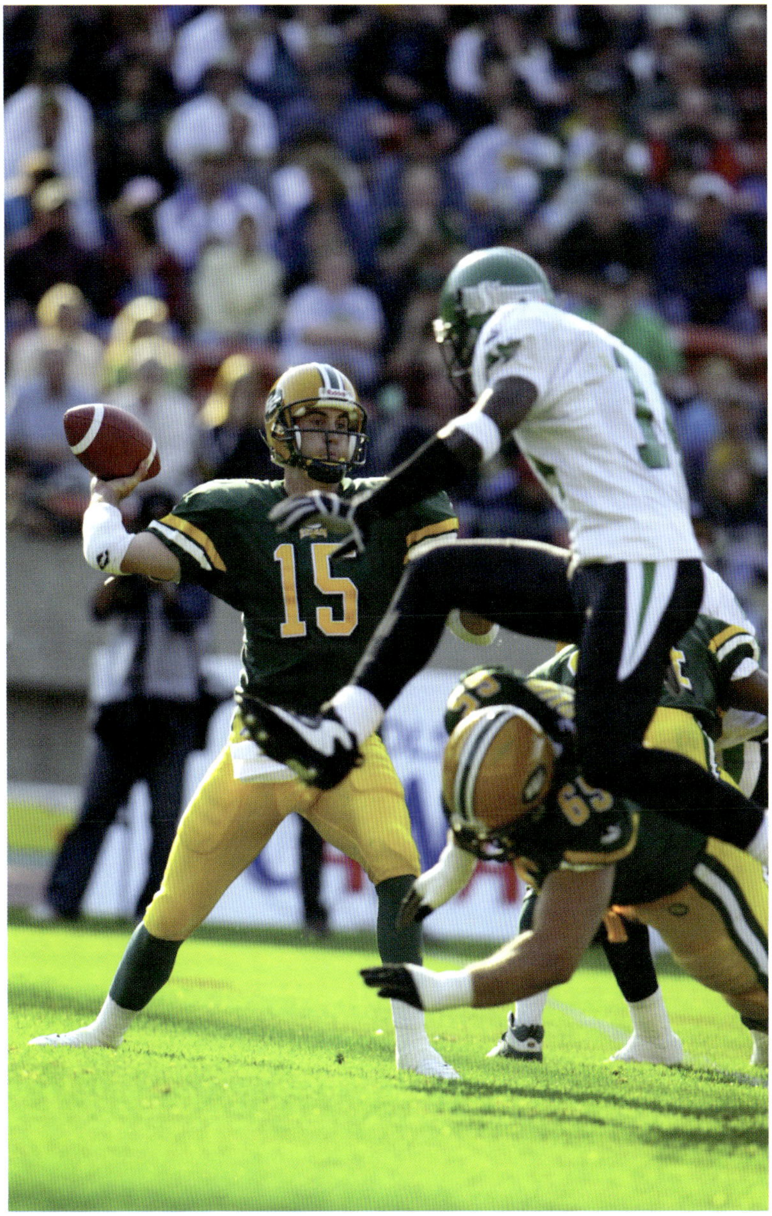

Ricky Ray gets ready to fire another strike.

Time for the Battle of Alberta.

The Calgary Stampeders were 2–8. Quarterback Marcus Crandell was hurt most of the time, and Coach Jim Barker was under pressure to start the owner's son, Kevin Feterik. While the defense played

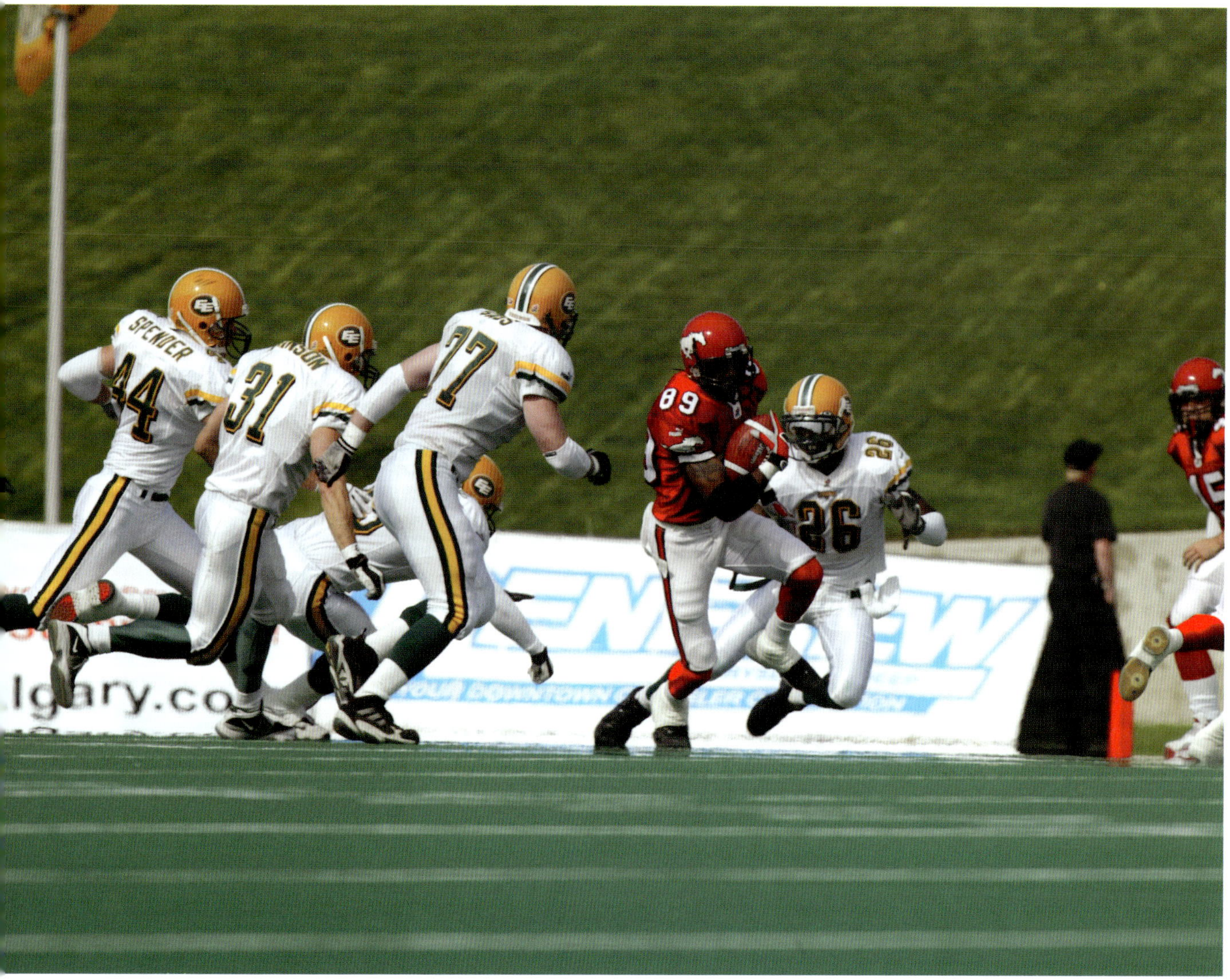

James Hundon takes it to the house.

reasonably well, the offense suffered from the revolving door syndrome at the most important position as well as a continuous string of injuries to key personnel like receivers Albert Connell and Darnell McDonald. Barker cut reliable veteran running back Kelvin Anderson in favor of the controversial Lawrence Phillips, who was later fired for insubordination. Owner Michael Feterik and Vice-Chairman and General Manager Fred Fateri angered Calgarians for running Wally Buono out of town and constantly interfering with the football operation. Dubbed the F-Troop by Calgary Herald columnist Bruce Dowbiggin, Feterik and Fateri, the California Carpetbaggers, were running a great franchise into the ground.

Although Calgarians had come to expect the bizarre on Labour Day, only a fool would have bet on the injury-riddled, trouble-plagued Stampeders to upset the mighty Eskimos. But upset them they did.

On their second possession of the game, Ricky Ray threw to

Vaughn for 15 yards, and Pringle ran for six. Sean Fleming was wide on a 42-yard field goal that speedster Wane McGarity returned 126 yards for a touchdown. Television replays would reveal the kick was good. But Calgary led 7–0. Following the kickoff, Ray marched the Eskimos 54 yards in seven plays. This time Fleming was credited with a 30-yard field goal. The Stamps kicked a single to end the scoring in the opening quarter.

Edmonton responded with a nine-play, 75-yard drive with Ray diving one yard into the end zone at the 36-second mark of the second quarter, giving the Eskimos a 10–8 lead. Mark McLoughlin kicked the Stamps back in front with a 31-yard field goal. Playing his best game of the year, Crandell drove his team 82 yards in four plays for a touchdown. The big strike was a 51-yard pass-and-run to McGarity that brought the ball to the Eskimo 31. Three plays later Don Blair made a great catch in the end zone for the major score. Calgary punter Duncan O'Mahoney added a single four minutes later.

Starting at his 35, Ray threw to Scott Robinson for five yards and to Vaughn for 15. He hit Tucker for a gain of 24 yards and Troy Mills for 14. On the next play, Ray was intercepted by Otis Floyd in the end zone. At halftime Calgary was up 19–10.

The battle seesawed back and forth during the third quarter. The Eskimos shut Calgary down but could only come up with a field goal and safety touch. After 45 minutes the Stampeders were still in the lead 19–15. Not for long.

On the first play of the fourth quarter, Ray and Tucker combined for a 64-yard pass-and-run to the end zone. Edmonton led 22–19. But, again, not for long. The Stampeders' James Hundon returned Fleming's kickoff 102 yards for a touchdown. Later, backed up on their one-yard line, the Esks closed out the scoring by giving up a safety touch. The shocking final score was Calgary 28, Edmonton 22. Environment Canada reported that Hell had frozen over.

As they boarded the bus to head for home, the Eskimos were 7–4 and tied with Winnipeg for second place. They would not taste defeat again until the last game of the regular season.

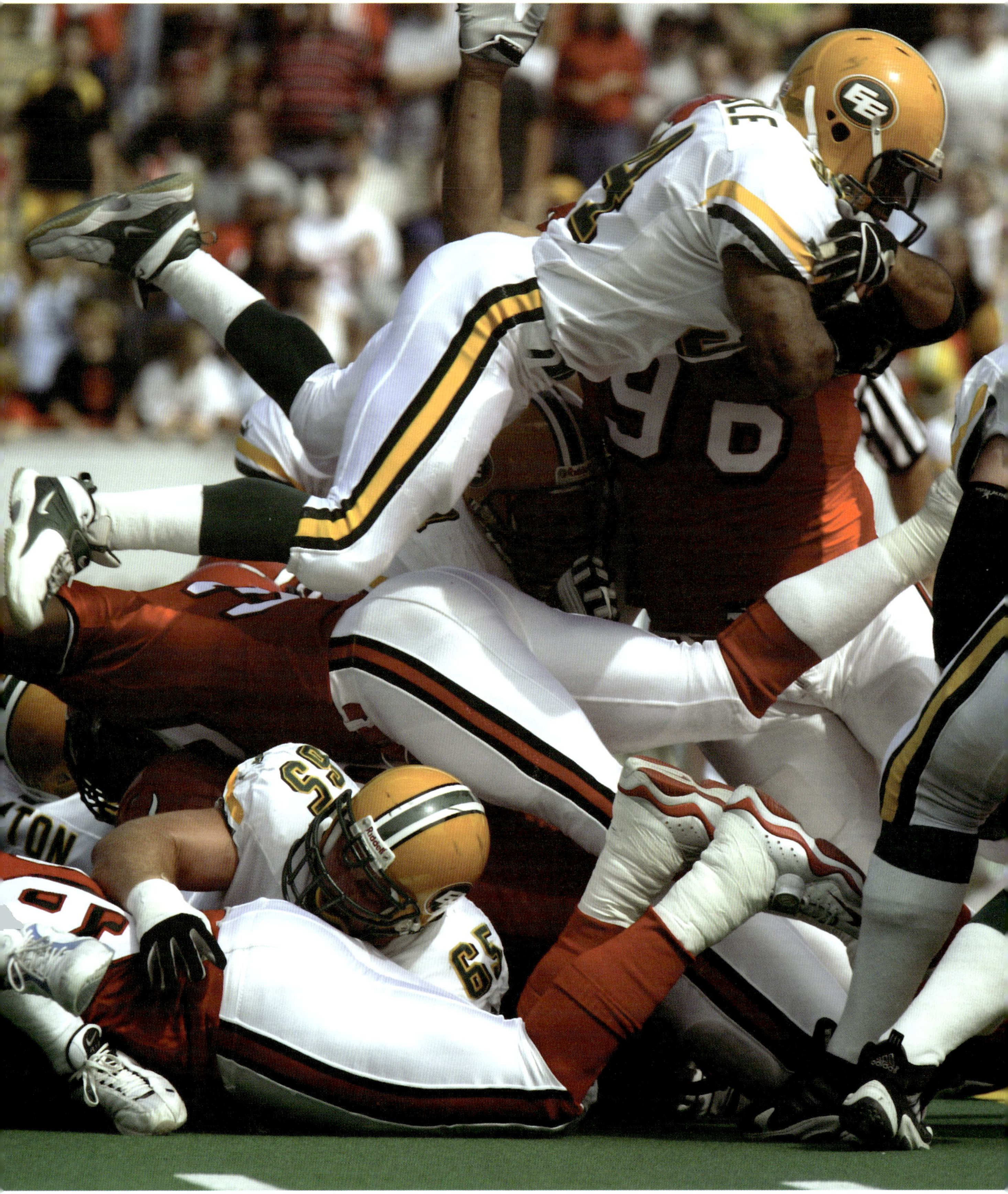
96
65
TON
Riddell

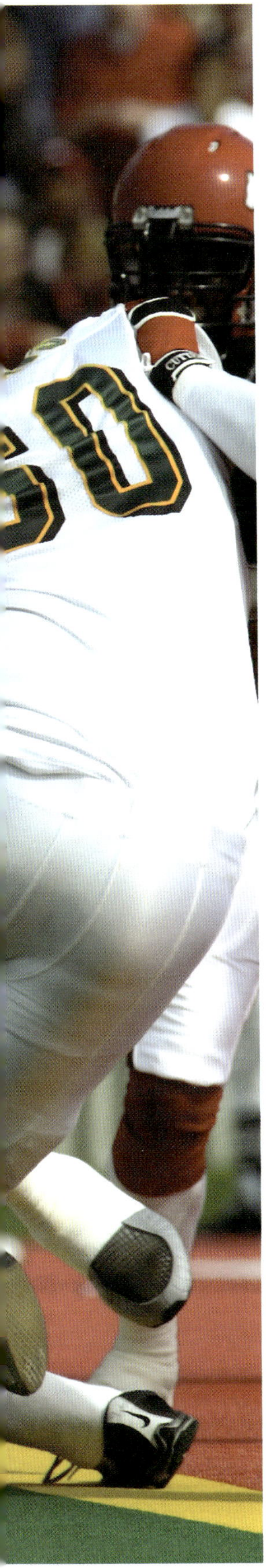

Labour Day in Calgary, the Battle of Alberta. I hear ya knockin', but ya can't come in. No. 6 Garrett Smith keeps Mike Pringle out of the end zone despite the best efforts of Kevin Lefsrud, No. 65, and Chris Morris, No. 60.

Chapter 4

When Autumn Leaves Turn to Gold

THE DRIVE FOR THE CUP

USUALLY, THE BIGGEST CROWD OF THE SEASON TO FILL THE stands at Commonwealth Stadium is the Friday night rematch against the Stampeders following the Labour Day Classic in Calgary. With two exceptions since 1969, Calgary has entertained the Eskimos at McMahon Stadium on Labour Day. Beginning in 1989, the Alberta rivals have met again the following Friday night in the provincial capital. In the 15-year history of the home-and-home series, Edmonton has swept four times, Calgary twice. Nine times, including 2003, they split.

The historic rivalry between the two great cities is enhanced each year by the Eskimos' promotion that allows a child in free on a parent's ticket. The Eskimos have always had the best and brightest marketing department in the country. They know that to remain prosperous and competitive they have to keep the people coming, and that means appealing to each new generation. Hooking young people on the CFL and green and gold is the secret of their success.

Certainly, winning helps as well. The Eskimos have only had eight losing seasons in their 55-year history. But given the community's record for supporting cultural and athletic events, it is very likely that the club would still lead the CFL in attendance, no matter where they placed in the standings. During the dynasty years, when it was almost

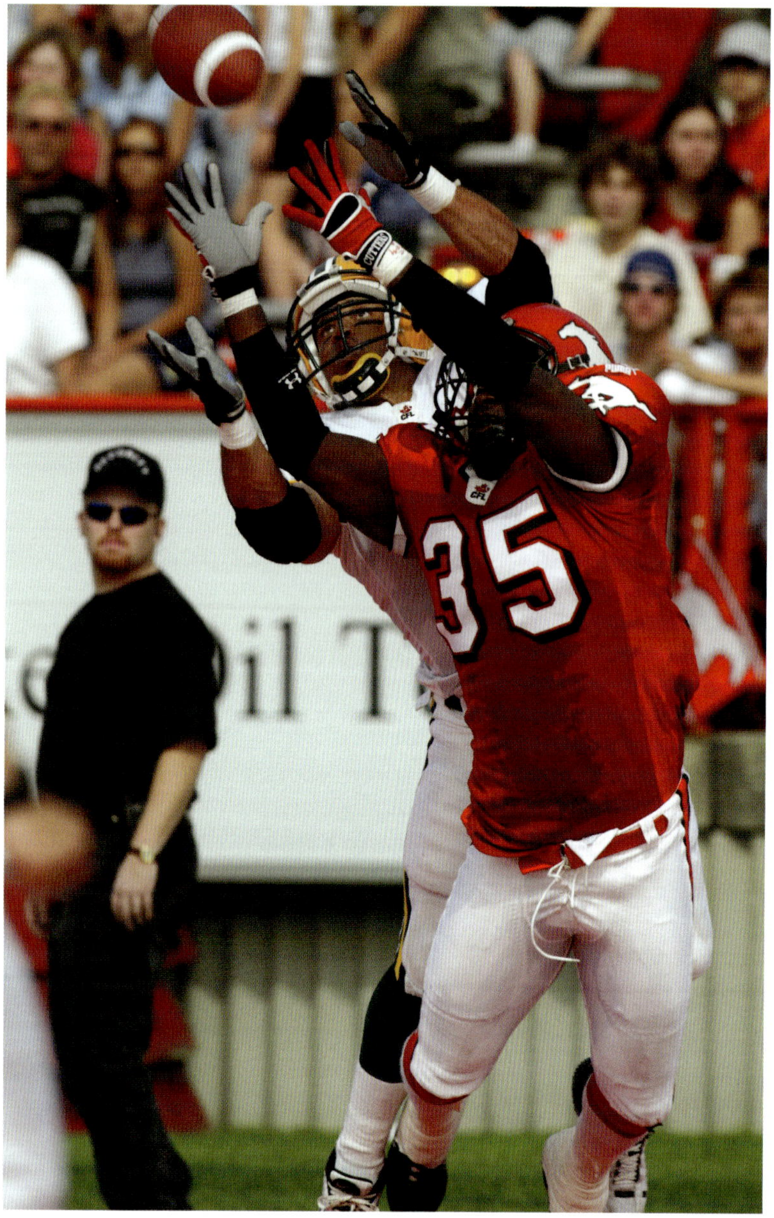

Otis Floyd makes a key interception at his 17-yard line to preserve the Calgary lead on Labour Day.

impossible to get into a game if you weren't a season-ticket holder, club PR guru Quincy Moffat was asked why he continued to have contests such as the one where the section that cheers the loudest gets a free barbecue.

"You have to make hay while the sun shines," he replied with a smile. "The day might come when you don't have a Warren Moon or Dan Kepley, when you're not winning the Grey Cup every year and you want your fans to remember how well they were treated so they'll come back."

The Eskimos still haven't experienced hard times on the field, but the CFL has gone through some pretty lean years. Yet Edmontonians kept coming to the ballpark. This blue collar yet cosmopolitan town is the City of Champions because of the people who live there.

A new stadium and CFL record for a regular season game was set September 5, 2003, when 62,444 fans filed into one of the finest football venues in North America. That eclipsed the mark of 61,481 set the year before when the Esks beat the Stamps 45–11.

After their embarrassing defeat down south, Mike Pringle and friends were determined there would be no loss this time. Edmonton opened the scoring nine and a half minutes into the first quarter when Troy "The Man Who Does Everything" Mills took a Ricky Ray pass 13 yards to the end zone. The Esks found the end zone three times in quarter number two, with touchdowns by Pringle, Scott Robinson and Jason Tucker. Pringle ran 61 yards to pay dirt two minutes into the second half. Sean Fleming added a 17-yard field goal in the fourth quarter. Final score: Edmonton 38, Calgary 0. A pall of gloom fell over the Stampede city once again.

Pringle had an exceptional

evening, carrying the mail 22 times for 148 yards and two touchdowns. Ray was sensational again, completing 22 of 27 passes for 266 yards and two TDs. Unusual for the young star, he had two picked off. Winston October caught 10 passes for 92 yards, Terry Vaughn five for 91. Singor Mobley was a whirling dervish on defense, making two interceptions and four tackles.

Two-thirds of the way through the season, the Eskimos sat alone in second place with eight wins and four losses, two points behind the Winnipeg Blue Bombers. The Lions and Roughriders were another game in back. Edmonton ranked fourth in rushing, third in passing and second in total offense. Third in passing behind Anthony Calvillo and Dave Dickenson, Ricky Ray had completed 233 of 342 passes for 2,974 yards and 23 touchdowns. He had been intercepted eight times. His 68.1 percent completion rate was three tenths of a point behind Medicine Hat's favorite son-in-law, Dave Dickenson. Ray was second in passing efficiency to the B.C. pivot. Both Calvillo and Dickenson were gnarly old veterans. The downy-cheeked Ray was blazing an incredible trail at the tender age of 24.

Edmonton's Terry Vaughn was second to Montreal's Jermaine Copeland in receiving with 69 grabs for 1,038 yards, the record-setting ninth consecutive season Vaughn surpassed the 1,000-yard mark. Because Ray spread the ball around, keeping all his receivers happy, there was a considerable drop for Ed Hervey, who caught 44 balls for 572 yards. Jason Tucker had 32 receptions for 558 yards. Ricky Walters, Scott Robinson, Troy Mills, Mike Pringle and, newly arrived from Regina, former Eskimo Quincy Jackson also contributed in the receiving department. It was impossible for enemy defenses to double-team a Vaughn

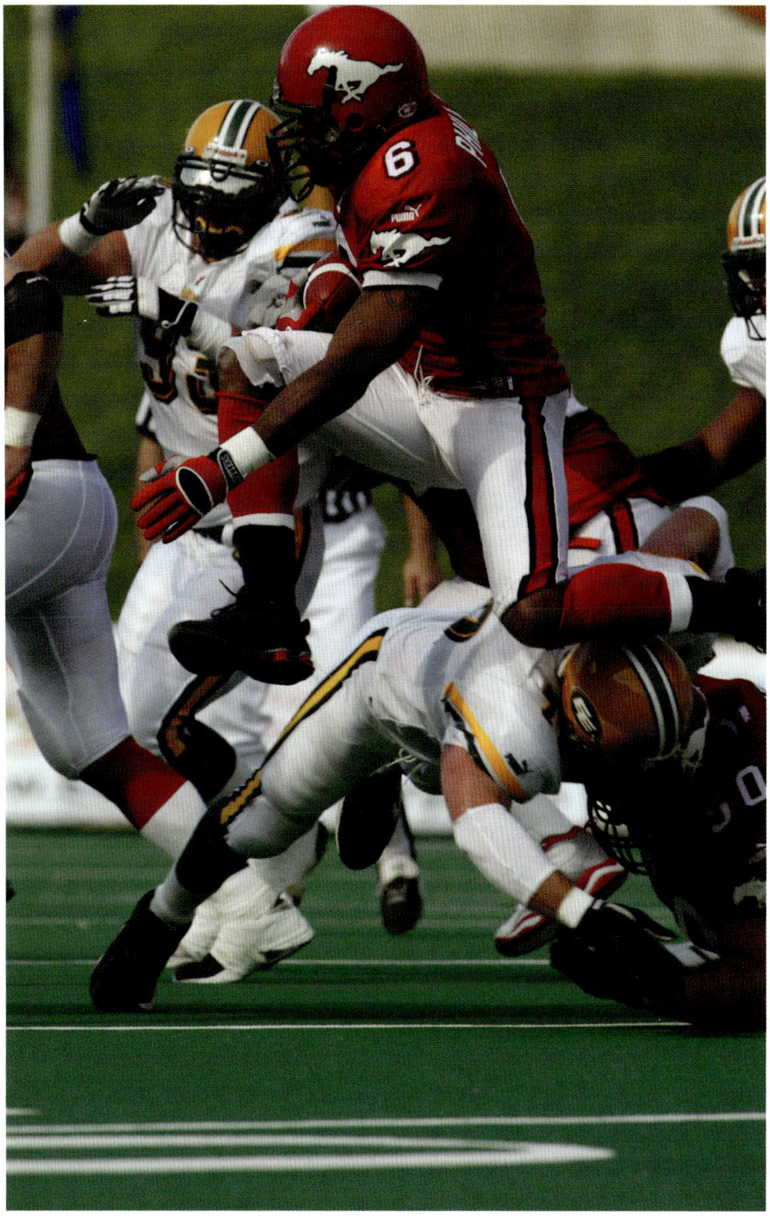

Lawrence Philips slips away from Steve Charbonneau for a 25-yard gain.

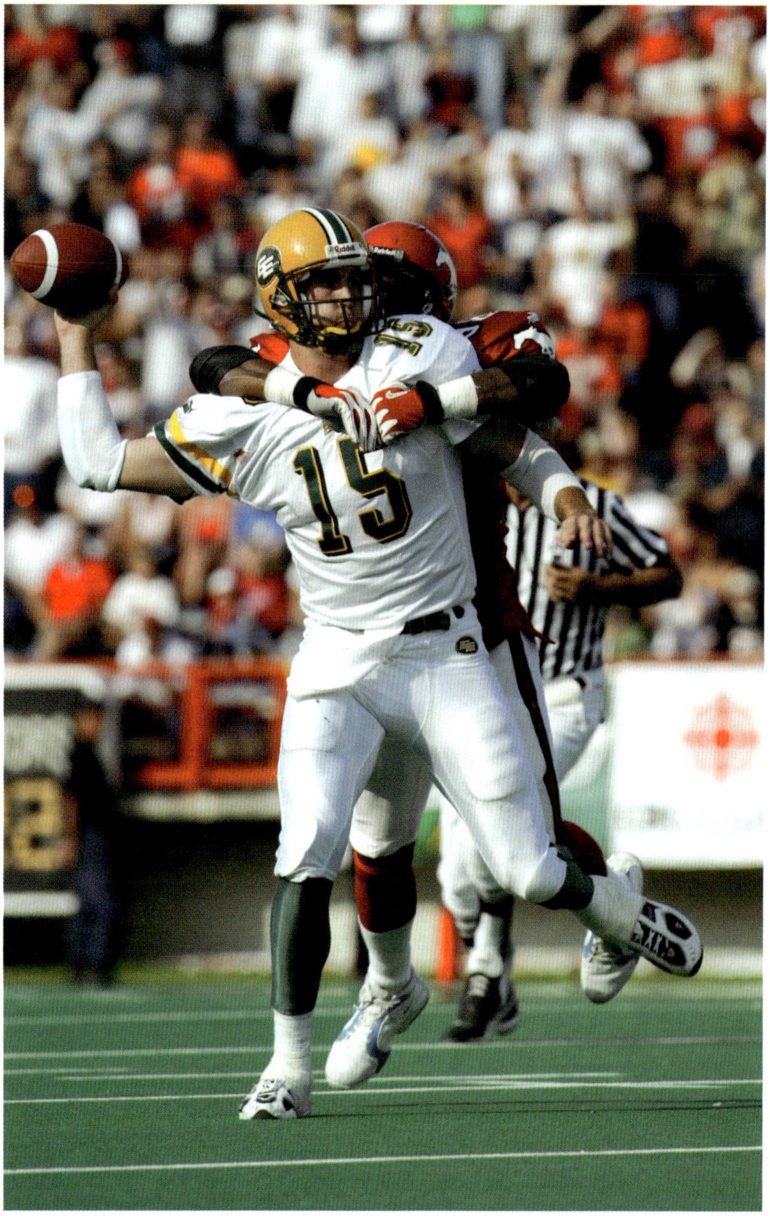

Ricky Ray pressured by George White.

or Tucker and shut the Eskimos down. Tom Higgins had too many weapons at his disposal.

Mike Pringle was certainly one of them, justifying the faith the Eskimo organization showed in signing the running back who had been out for a year with what is usually a career-ending injury and who celebrated his 36th birthday on October 1. Old Man River Pringle just kept rolling along, second in rushing with 1,032 yards, the eighth time he passed the season century mark. He also had 201 receiving yards.

Strengthened by the return of Kelvin Kinney from Toronto, the defense was in fine form, leading the nation in pass defense and average yards surrendered per game, even though they were only sixth in quarterback sacks. They were second to B.C. in points against, giving up an average of 18.8 points per game. They were third in the Giveaway–Takeaway category with a +7.

But old habits die hard. Despite making every effort to improve, only Hamilton was worse in the fumble department while only the Blue Bombers gave up more penalty yards. The worst offense came on Labour Day in Calgary when Ed Hervey was ejected for hitting line judge Brent Buchko with his helmet while taking a swing at Stampeder cornerback Davis Sanchez. Hervey was suspended for one game, first by the Eskimos who made it clear such behavior would not be tolerated and then by the league.

No single individual stood out on defense. Collectively they did a great job honoring the team's promotional slogan, "Defend The Turf." They did that as well or better than anybody. The formidable front four consisted of Kelvin Kinney, Albert Reese, Steve Charbonneau and Rahim Abdullah, who showed no ill effects from his bout with Ephedrine. Linebackers Singor Mobley, Kelvin Powell, A.J.

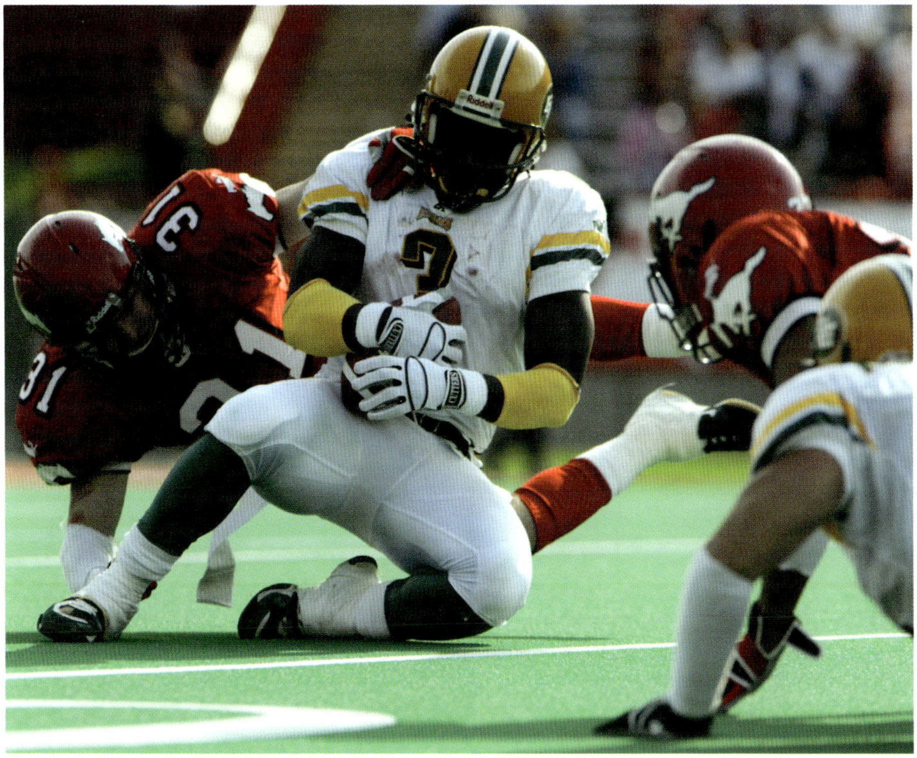

I've got it! I've got it! Terry Vaughn makes a great diving catch for 13 yards.

Gass and Rob Grant had a mean streak that intimidated the opposition. And the secondary of Malcolm Frank, Shannon Garrett, Quincy Coleman, Donny Brady and Darrel Crutchfield, a team weakness in 2002, had become one of the best in the nation.

Special teams were solid.

The heart of the schedule lay ahead. Between September 13 and October 25, the Eskimos would play B.C. and Winnipeg twice, as well as Les Alouettes in Montreal. The head-to-head match-ups with the Lions and Blue Bombers would determine first place in the West.

Out in what Jack Gotta used to call "The Big Tent," the Lions and Eskimos clashed for the first time during the regular season. In an exciting game before 27,070 fans at B.C. Place, the Lions opened the scoring five minutes in when Dave Dickenson hit his favorite target, Geroy Simon, for a 26-yard touchdown. Ricky Ray struck back with two first-quarter TDs, a seven-yard pass to Troy Mills and a nine-yarder to Winston October. Sean Fleming booted two field goals in the second quarter. The Lions responded with a Kelvin Anderson touchdown before Curtis Head closed out the scoring in the first half with a 49-yard field goal. Edmonton led 20–17.

Considering the aerial show Dickenson and Ray were staging, the third quarter was relatively quiet. Fleming conceded a safety touch, Head kicked a 34-yard field goal and Ray connected with Ed Hervey for a touchdown. At the end of the quarter the Eskimos still led 27–22.

Sixteen seconds into the final fifteen minutes, Simon made a superb catch for a 39-yard major. Dickenson and Simon then teamed up for a two-point conversion, putting B.C. back into the lead 30–27. Simon had an incredible night with 10 catches for 238 yards. After an excellent return, Ray and Hervey answered back two minutes and 38 seconds later with a touchdown of their own. The Esks hung on to win 34–30. The Lions were their own worst enemy, turning the ball over six times. Still, as Hervey said after the game, "We came in here with a playoff mentality, and we pulled it out."

Rickie Ray was good on 28 of 36 passes for 339 yards and four touchdowns while throwing no interceptions. The well-rested and repentant Hervey caught eight throws for 126 yards and twelve points. Pringle picked up 97 yards rushing. Donny Brady picked off the Lion's pivot twice.

Back home against the Renegades, Ray got off to a sizzling start, completing his first 10 passes and running up a 35–7 lead by the half. After throwing a touchdown strike to Ricky Walters and capping off a long drive by diving into the end zone from the one, Edmonton led 14–7. The Eskimos scored three touchdowns in less than two minutes, including a 22-yard strike to Ed Hervey and a spectacular 64-yard pass-and-run to the same receiver. With ten seconds left in the half, Rob Grant recovered a fumble on the kickoff and took it to the house.

As was their wont all season, the Eskimos, enjoying a 28-point lead, let up in the second half, being outscored by the Renegades 26–10. It didn't matter, though; the final score was Edmonton 45, Ottawa 33. Ray was 21 for 24 for 339 yards. His 87.5 percent completion rate matched a Joe Paopao outing for the Lions in 1979 as the third-best single-game mark in CFL history. The record is 90.5 percent (on 19 for 21 passing) set by Edmonton's Tom Wilkinson against Ottawa on August 19, 1974, and equaled by Danny McManus for Hamilton against Winnipeg on October 10, 1999.

Donny Brady turned in another sparkling performance with two interceptions.

With the win, the Eskimos were 10–4, two points up on Winnipeg, four on the third-place Lions, and six on the Roughriders. B.C. was coming to town. A victory over Wally Buono's Leos would go a long way in eliminating them from the race for first place.

Ray took care of business early, throwing to Terry Vaughn in the end zone less than five minutes after the opening kickoff. Before the quarter ended, Winston October ran 12 yards to the end zone to increase the Eskimo lead to 14. Pringle added a score in the second quarter. The Lions didn't get on the scoreboard until the last minute of the third quarter when Jason Clermont caught a touchdown pass from

Dickenson. Ray and Jason Tucker replied early in the fourth quarter. The convert was no good. The final score before a crowd of 44,432 was Edmonton 27, B.C. 7. With the win Edmonton clinched a playoff spot for the 32nd straight year.

Terry Vaughn led the way with 142 yards and a touchdown on 11 receptions. Donny Brady was everywhere, making five tackles and forcing two fumbles.

Off to Montreal, where the Eskimos hadn't won in 20 years. At 12–2, Don Matthews' Alouettes had already clinched first place in the East. Adding to the drama was Mike Pringle's return to the city he played in for seven years.

Ray and Hervey opened the scoring with a 10-yard touchdown at 5:10 of the first quarter. Matt Kellett responded with a field goal, as well as another one in the second frame. Fleming split the uprights from 19 yards out, and Pringle made a successful return to Percival Molson Memorial Stadium by running over from the one. At halftime the Eskimos had a surprisingly easy 17–6 lead. A Fleming field goal made it 20–6 after three quarters of play.

Never one to kick an opponent when he's down, the Eskimos let the Als back in it and had to hang on for a 20–19 win. They were six points up on Winnipeg and B.C. with a week off to prepare themselves for the stretch run.

That began on October 17 when the Bombers came to town, now trailing Edmonton by four points in the standings. If Winnipeg could sweep the season-ending series with the Eskimos, they would finish first. The Green and Gold weren't about to let that happen.

Over 45,000 fans watched the Eskimos clinch first place by knocking off the Bombers 41–32. The game started off with a bang when Mike Bradley from Waterloo ran the opening kickoff 92 yards to the end zone. Winnipeg answered soon after with a Mike Sellers touchdown. The two teams battled back and forth on a gorgeous evening, providing the huge crowd with wonderful entertainment.

Pat Barnes had replaced the ailing Khari Jones at quarterback and played very well for Winnipeg, showing poise and resilience in the face of a ferocious Eskimo defense. Ricky Ray was brilliant for the Eskimos, time and time again exploiting the pass rush by dumping off to Mike Pringle and Troy Mills.

With first place in the bag, the Esks headed for frigid Winnipeg, where they blew a lead and lost their last game of the season, 34–30. Winnipeg's win and B.C.'s loss to Saskatchewan created a three-way tie for second place at 11–7. Once the tiebreakers were employed, B.C. was placed fourth and would go east to face the Argonauts while the second-place Blue Bombers would host the third-place Roughriders in the Western semifinal. All snug in their beds at home in the Igloo, the 13–5 Eskimos awaited the winner.

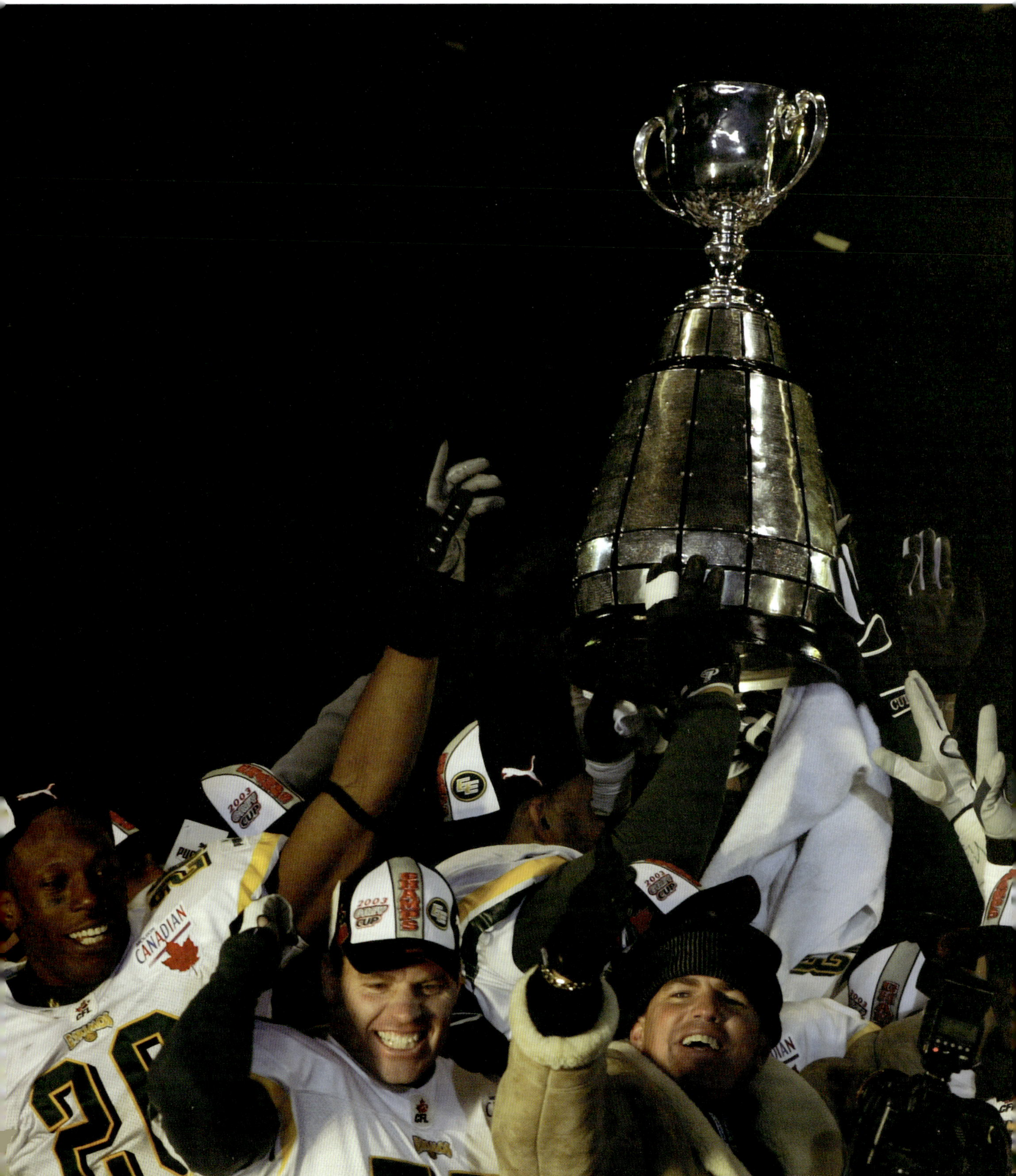
2003
CHAMPS
CANADIAN

Chapter 5

Grey Cup Green & Gold

GREY CUP 2003

For the first time in a decade, the Grey Cup comes back to the City of Champions.

AFTER DROPPING THE LAST GAME OF THE REGULAR SEASON in Winnipeg, Ricky Ray found the silver lining in the dark cloud. "We haven't lost since Labour Day," he said, "so maybe this is a good reminder about how bad it feels to lose and it'll give us extra motivation going into the Western final."

During the regular season they had lost to and defeated both Saskatchewan and Winnipeg. It didn't matter to most of the Eskimos who they played, as long as they won and made it back to the Grey Cup. It did matter to most of them who came out of the East: to a man they wanted to play Montreal.

Because of television policy, the indoor Eastern game was shown in the afternoon, the Western semifinal at night. The same process would be repeated the following week. Winter had come to the prairies the last week of October, and by kickoff time at 5:00 P.M. local time, the temperature with the wind chill factored in was -20°C.

Both teams had 11–7 records, but the Bombers had beaten the Roughriders both times they met during the regular season. Their great rivalry in Canadian sport that goes back 91 years, and Winnipeg kicker Troy Westwood stoked the fires further by first of all calling Saskatchewan folks banjo picking in-breds and then later "apologized" by saying most

Saskatchewan people didn't know how to play the banjo. Although it was obviously said in fun (Westwood's family, after all, is from the Land of Living Skies), the Roughriders were not amused.

Spurred on by the Tractor Factor (over 3,500 Rider fans made the trek to Canad Inns Stadium), the Roughies socked it to the Blue Bombers in convincing fashion. If the Eastern semifinal between the Lions and the Argonauts resembled a ballet, the Western semifinal played in frigid conditions on a frozen field was good old-fashioned smash-mouth prairie football.

The game promised a showdown between the best running attack in the league, that of Saskatchewan, versus the top run defense which had yielded only 72.8 yards per game. The Riders' Kenton Keith carried the ball 14 times for 130 of his team's 200 yards rushing total, as well as scoring three touchdowns. His performance was necessary to overcome Nealon Greene's anemic passing performance: 5 for 15, 93 yards and a touchdown. That major was scored by Matt Dominguez, who went 55 yards to the end zone, meaning Greene completed only four more passes for a grand total of 38 yards the rest of the way.

Saskatchewan led 17–0 at the end of the first quarter and 20–8 at the half. With the injured Khari Jones in for the injured Pat Barnes, the Bombers rallied in the third quarter, closing the gap to 20–18. All they could muster thereafter was a field goal while the Riders added two TDs and a three-pointer to win going away, 37–21. On to Edmonton.

The Green and White were surprisingly confident going into Edmonton, even though they had only won twice at Commonwealth Stadium over the last 10 years, including the 1997 Western final. They were determined to reward their long-suffering faithful fans by playing in their Grey Cup at Taylor Field one week later. The possibility of that seemed remote before the season began and when the team slumped badly in August. But after winning five in a row, including games in Calgary, Vancouver and Winnipeg, the Rider nation dared to dream the impossible dream. Still, the teams matched up rather well.

The Eskimos were third in total offense with 382 yards per game, Saskatchewan fourth with 359. The Riders were first in rushing, important at this time of the year, Edmonton fourth. Mike Pringle accounted for two-thirds of his team's rushing total. If Saskatchewan could shut him down they way they did Charles Roberts in Winnipeg, they would force Ricky Ray to attack their strength, which was pass defense.

The Eskimos were third in passing, Saskatchewan eighth. The Esks' offensive line allowed the fewest sacks in the league, 25, but the Riders were second at 27. The

Roughies threw the fewest interceptions, 13; Edmonton was close behind with 17. Saskatchewan took fewer penalties while the Eskimos continued to be somewhat undisciplined.

Defensively, the Riders were second against the pass, Edmonton fourth. At stopping the run, Edmonton was fourth, Saskatchewan sixth. The visitors surrendered the fewest touchdown passes.

Edmonton's Giveaway–Takeaway rating was +10, Saskatchewan's +9. Edmonton recorded 44 sacks and 24 interceptions, Saskatchewan 40 and 22. Special teams? Both had superb return games and cover teams. Paul McCallum and Sean Fleming were outstanding veteran kickers.

Unlike the Lions, who were doomed when Dave Dickenson couldn't play in the Eastern semifinal, the Riders and Eskimos were deep at quarterback and wouldn't miss a beat if the starter was injured. In fact, as it turned out, it would have been a blessing in disguise for the Roughriders if Greene had gone down in the first quarter.

The game-playing began long before the kickoff. It has been Eskimo practice to keep visiting teams from Commonwealth Stadium until their pre-game warm-up. While Hugh Campbell has always insisted it was to protect the "best natural grass field" in Canada, opponents suspected it was to put them at a disadvantage both physically and psychologically in terms of choosing the best footwear for the conditions. This time Rider Head Coach Danny Barrett and GM Roy Shivers did an end-run on the home team by asking and receiving permission from the CFL to go on the field the day before the game.

Attempting an end-run of their own, the Eskimos Chief Operating Officer Rick LeLacheur and

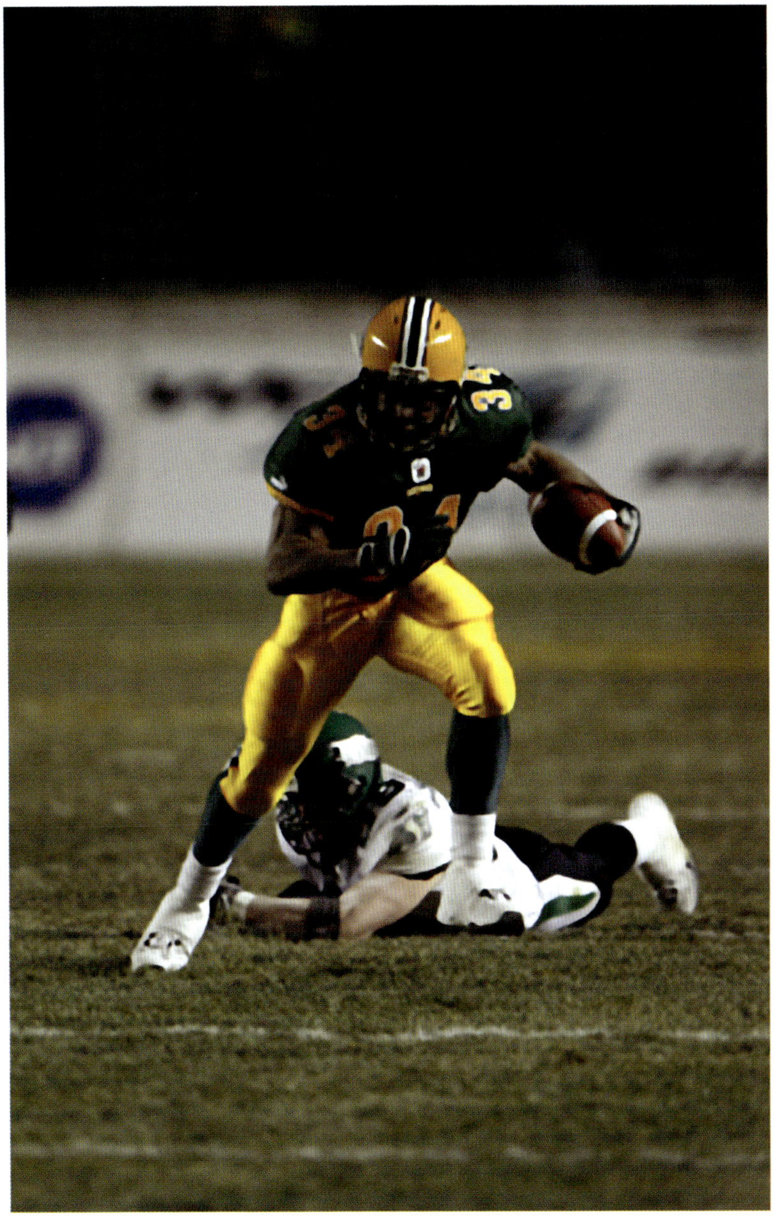

Mike Pringle making the Roughriders eat his dust in the Western final.

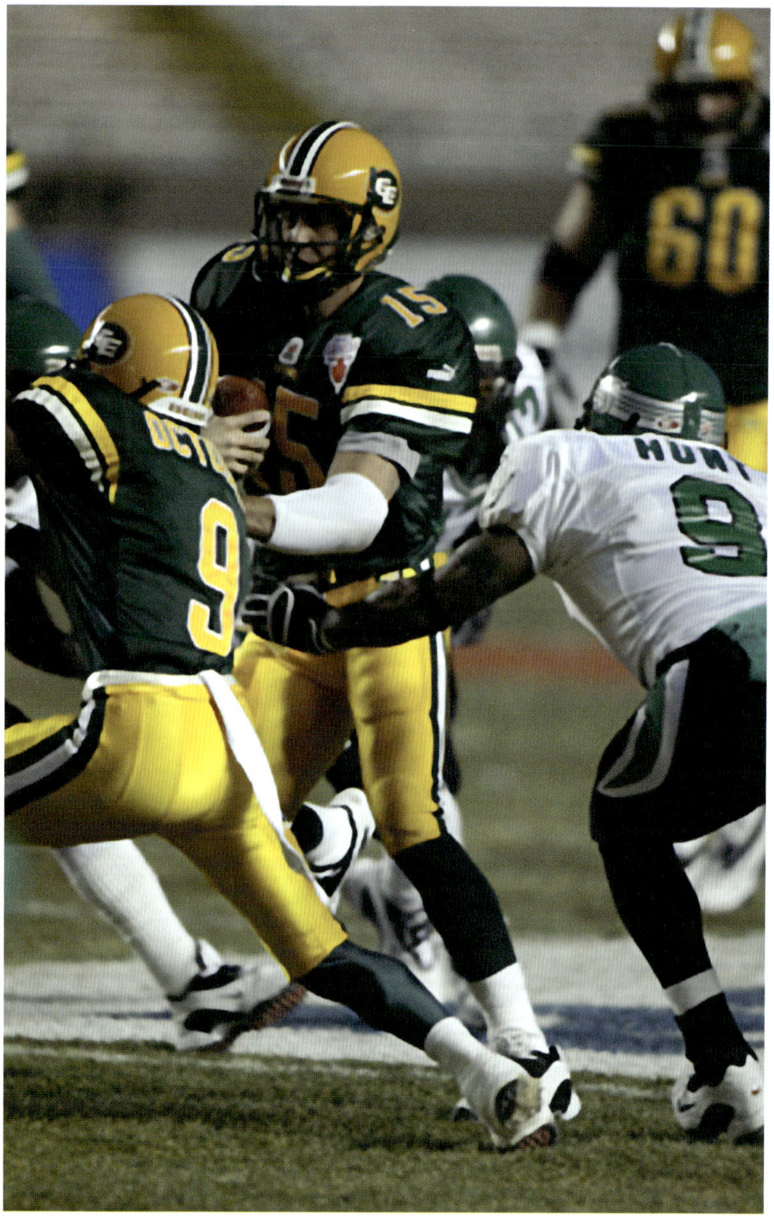

The Roughriders Reggie Hunt wraps up Ricky Ray.

Defensive Back Coach Rick Campbell removed all the standing advertising signs from the south end zone, intending to keep the Riders behind the goal line while they tested the turf.

Barrett would have none of it. "We're going to adhere to everything we talked about," he informed LeLacheur. "I talked to the league." At least Saskatchewan would win the mind games.

That's all they'd win. Despite some last-minute heroics by Rider quarterback Kevin Glenn, the Eskimos were in control from wire to wire. It was the brilliance of second-year man Ricky Ray versus the ineptitude of six-year veteran Nealon Greene.

When the Western final began at 5:00 P.M. local time, the temperature hovered near zero. Among the 40,081 paying customers were thousands dressed in green and white.

Despite the Eskimos' total domination in the opening quarter, they could only manage two Sean Fleming singles. The second quarter wasn't much better, but given airtight protection by his offensive line, Ray finally put together a nine-play, 85-yard touchdown drive. The big plays were 30- and 33-yard passes to Vaughn and October. Mike Pringle picked up 13 yards on the ground and 11 through the air. With second-and-goal from the eight, Ray rolled right and found Troy Mills open in the end zone.

The ensuing Saskatchewan possession was a comedy of errors. Chris Szarka returned the kickoff 10 yards to his 47. Kenton Keith was thrown for a one-yard loss. Greene threw to Corey Grant for 19 yards. Dorian Boose then nailed the Riders' quarterback six yards behind the line. Greene replied with a 33-yard strike to Jason French, bringing the ball to the Eskimo 18. In the shotgun formation, Greene bobbled the snap and

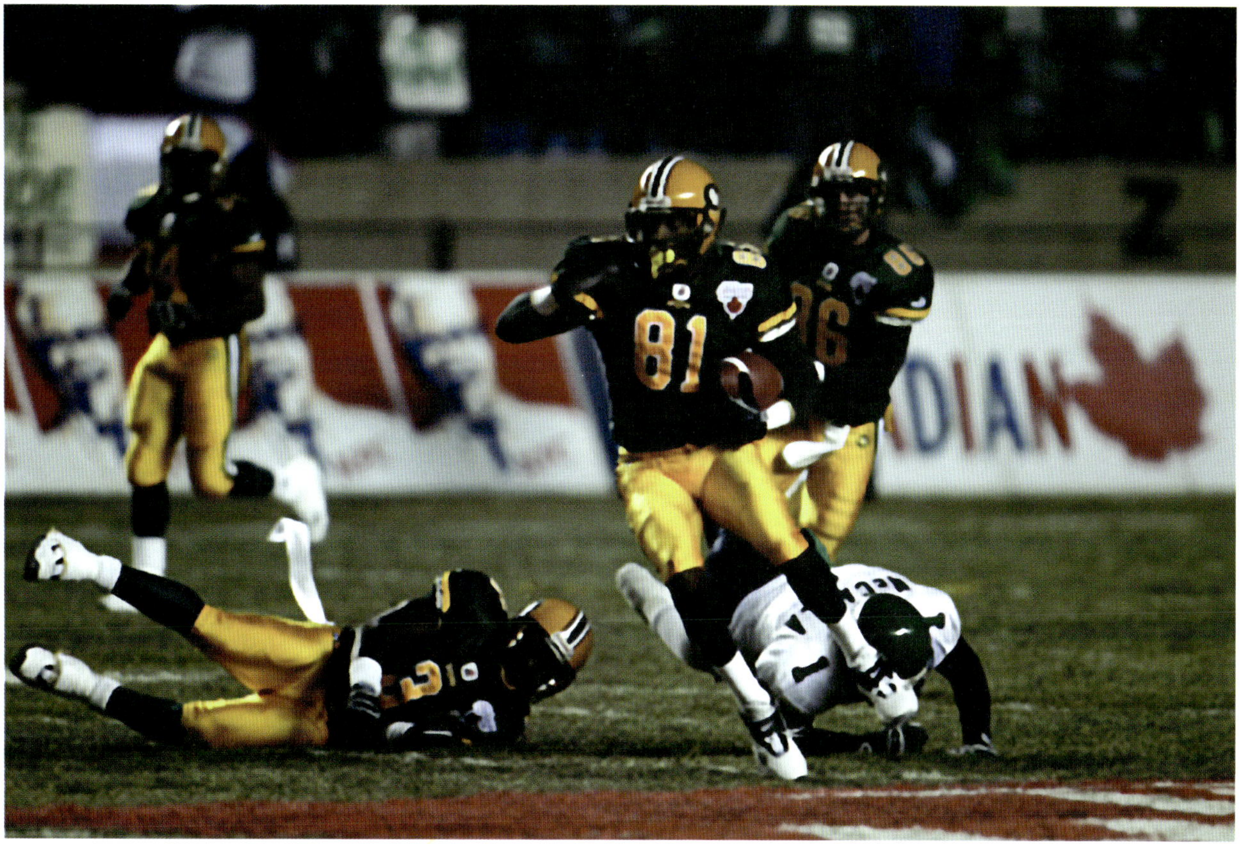

was tackled back at the 32-yard line. Greene completed a 28-yard pass to Keith but the Roughriders were called for holding. Grant almost made a circus catch in the end zone. Edmonton was offside, making it second-and-29 from the 37. Kelvin Kinney sacked Greene back at the 43. Paul McCallum punted for a single.

Then it was Edmonton's turn. After moving 31 yards on two passes, Jason Tucker fumbled at the Rider 42. Terrence Melton returned it 48 yards to the enemy 20. Greene completed a 20-yard touchdown pass to Travis Moore that was nullified when Jamal Richardson was called for offensive interference. Two plays later, Brady intercepted Greene in the end zone.

At the half, Edmonton had 16 first downs to Saskatchewan's three. The Eskimos had 274 yards in total offense, the Riders 91. Nealon Greene was 4 for 10 and 66 yards while Ricky Ray completed 15 of 20 passes for 213 yards. The Roughriders' vaunted running attack was held to just 25 yards. Kenton Keith, who had ripped the Blue Bombers apart the week before, had two carries for three yards. It remains a mystery why Danny Barrett eschewed the run in favor of the pass.

While Greene was constantly under pressure, Ricky Ray had so much time he could have read War and Peace back there. He completed passes to eight different receivers, executing a brilliantly

After sewing up his finger, Ed Hervey takes a pass and heads up field.

conceived game plan by offensive coordinator Danny Maciocia. Still, thanks to the overworked Saskatchewan defense, the score was only 9–1.

The Riders' Paul McCallum made it 9–2 four minutes into the third quarter on another punt. Then Ricky Ray and Ed Hervey combined for a 69-yard pass-and-run for a touchdown. Before the half, Hervey had to leave because a finger was dislocated at a 90-degree angle with the bone piercing the skin. Hervey had it realigned and sewn up in the dressing room; he returned to the field just as McCallum was booting his single. No guts, no glory. Hervey had plenty of both.

Also back in action was Donny Brady, who had been leveled in the second quarter by Matt Dominguez' block. Brady still ached a week later.

On Edmonton's next possession, Ray marched his team 100 yards in 10 plays with Pringle going in from the two. With the score 23–2 and 2:16 left in the quarter, Danny Barrett finally sent Greene to the sideline in favor of Kevin Glenn. The day before, at the press conference, when questioned about Greene's poor play in Winnipeg, Barrett replied that Anthony Calvillo had won the Grey Cup the year before with a 35 percent completion rate.

Kevin Glenn would make things interesting.

But not before Ray capped off another 100-yard drive by scoring himself from the eight-yard line, an 11-play effort that took over five minutes off to the clock. With 9:22 remaining, and trailing 30–2, Kevin Glenn went to work. Utilizing Holmes, French, Moore, Keith and Szarka, Glenn took the Green and White 89 yards on 10 plays in three minutes and 41 seconds, Szarka doing the honors.

The two-point convert was good. It was two and out for Edmonton. Glenn then engineered a nine-play, 98-yard drive for the Riders' second major. Matt Dominguez scored the touchdown. This time the two-point attempt failed. The score was Edmonton 30, Saskatchewan 16, but only 56 seconds remained.

Successfully executing the short kickoff, the Riders scored a third TD on Glenn's quick passes and Szarka's one-yard plunge, making it 30–23. Eighteen seconds to go. Were the Roughriders about to pull off the greatest comeback in CFL history? It wasn't to be.

They recovered the short kickoff again, but Saskatchewan's Mike McCullough was called for interference. The Eskimos were going to the Grey Cup in Regina.

Tom Higgins was quietly ecstatic. "It is not easy to get back to the Grey Cup. Our players have been focused all year. We were able to finish in first place. We knew we only had to play a single game in order to get back to the Grey Cup, and all these things have fallen into place.

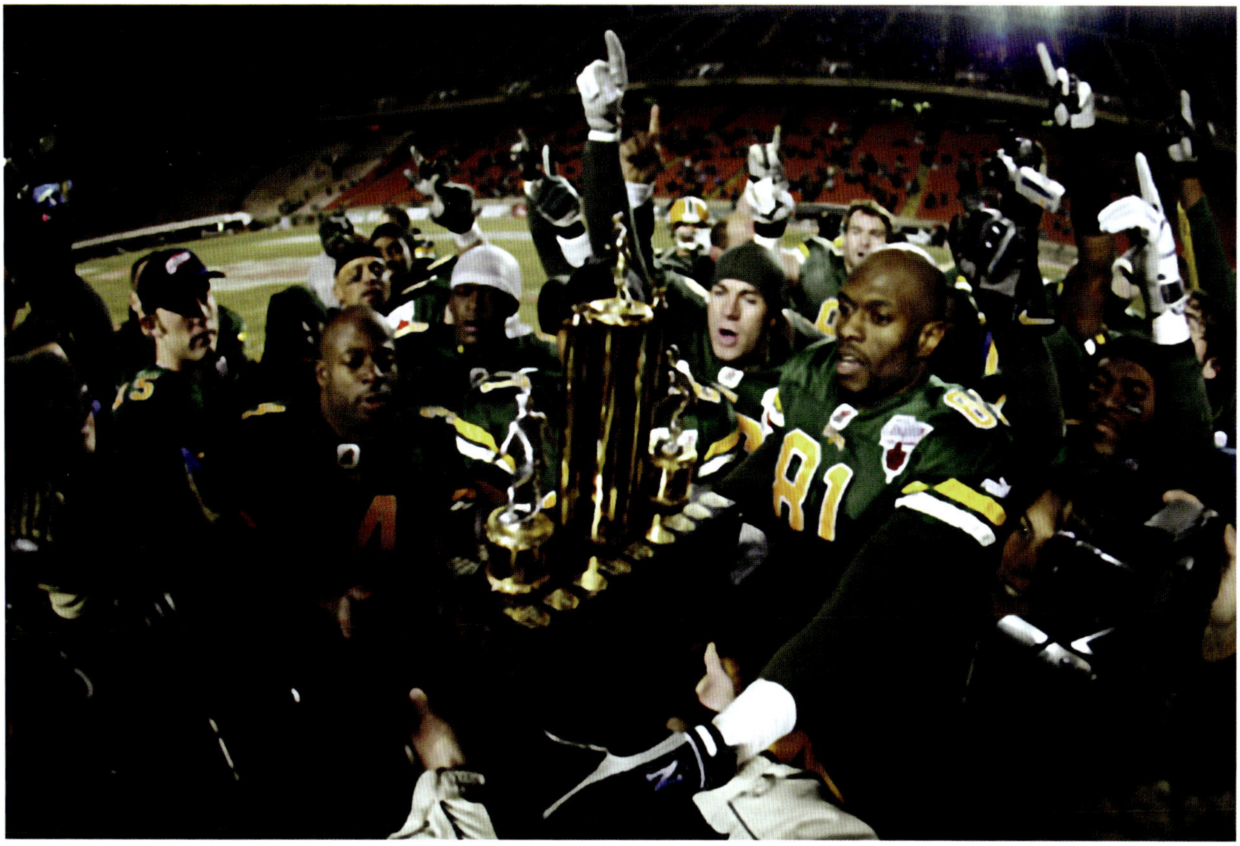

Ed Hervey and friends, Western Conference Champions.

"It has been a really fun, fun journey, and now the journey takes its final step, which is the Grey Cup. The bottom line is one team is going to be happy on Sunday and other will focus on next year. We like our chances."

When reminded that in three years he had gone from coaching his son's bantam team to his second berth in the Grey Cup, he laughed and replied, "We actually won a provincial championship with those little bantam kids. A championship is a championship. When you have a chance to be the best in Canada and put your name on a Grey Cup, that's pretty special."

Mike Pringle was almost at a loss for words. "I can't even explain how badly I wanted to get to the Grey Cup. I've got a couple of rings, and I know what it feels like to hoist that Cup up.

"What brings me the most pleasure is that so many people, so-called experts, said that Mike Pringle is done. Mike Pringle can't play football. There was some doubt, some people saying I couldn't recover from a knee injury, some people saying I was too old to play. I don't listen to people who are negative. I try to stay away from negative people. I know how hard I work. I know how hard I pray. I pray harder than I work."

Ricky Ray was analytical about the Western final. "In the first half, we had a hard time coming away with points. We did a better job in

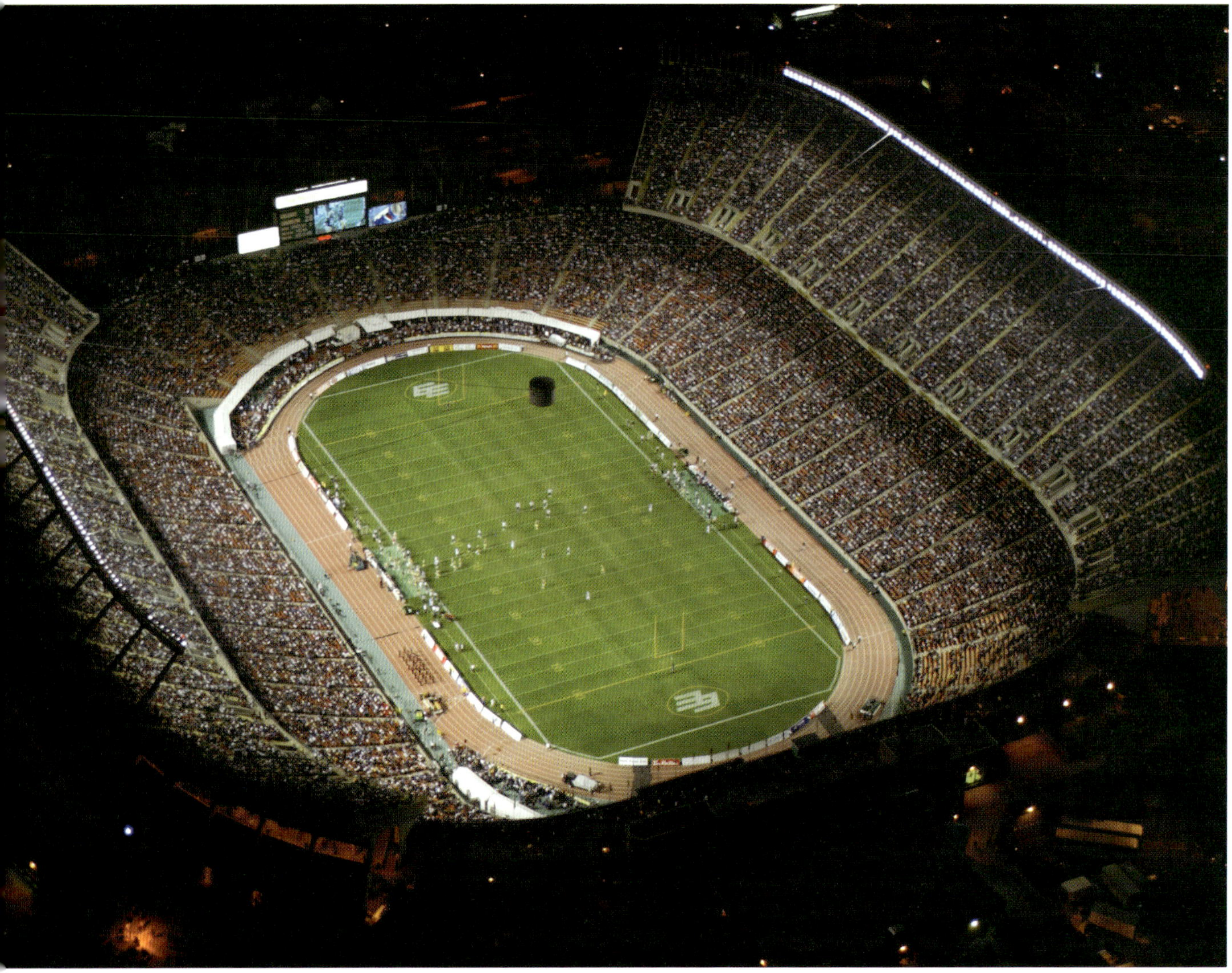

The stands are packed for the Western final. Happy Anniversay, Commonwealth Stadium.

the second half. We had big plays like the touchdown pass to Ed Hervey and converting an interference call into six points. We finished drives and finally shut the door on those guys."

He, too, looked forward with confidence to November 16. "You've got to go out and make plays, get field position, don't turn the ball over, execute the offense. If we are able to do those things, we'll have a pretty good shot."

Although he maintained he wasn't motivated to play well by the presence of NFL scouts in the press box, the fact that not a single Eskimo was up for a league award made him determined to prove that the Football Reporters of Canada were wrong.

"Certainly the best team in the West didn't have any final nominees. It just shows that we have a lot of good players on the team and nobody really stands out. Everybody just plays their role and goes out and does their job."

At that point Singor Mobley stuck his head in and yelled, "I don't know why he wasn't voted in as MVP of the league. He got robbed. We must be in Florida and need a recount. Recount!"

The Eskimos looked forward to playing Montreal.

"It makes for a nice story line to meet again in the Grey Cup," mused Higgins. "These are two very good football teams that finished first and have an opportunity to play for the Cup.

"All Grey Cups are special. People from all across the country come. They plan their vacations around it. Any Grey Cup that has ever been played on the prairies has always come off in my mind as one of the elite events because of the great volunteers we have out here. I can guarantee you that Regina will be ready for a great party. Two good football teams should culminate in a pretty good game to finish the football season."

Regina was ready for the 91st Grey Cup. With every hotel room booked over a year in advance, with thousands opening their homes to visitors, the good people of the Queen City were both party animals and perfect hosts. Entertainment venues were packed from Wednesday afternoon through Sunday night, and a great time was had by all.

While getting out and enjoying the atmosphere was certainly on the agenda, both teams knew why they were there and what was really important. Higgins looked ahead to Sunday.

"Montreal's a bit different than last year. They rely on throwing the football and we have a balanced attack. We now have a lot more players who have Grey Cup experience. They should be able to handle the pressure of being able to go back to the big game with all the media that's around and all the scrutiny that goes with it. They should feel pretty comfortable having done that before. A year ago in Edmonton they were under the microscope more than here in Regina. I know they are looking forward to it. We've put a couple of things together that we learned from last year: how to control the excitement, how to get through it. We'll be prepared and we'll put a very good product on the field."

Most pundits believed the game would be too close to call, although Las Vegas made the Eskimos a 3 1/2 point favorite. It would be an intriguing matchup.

"Alas, my love, you do me wrong to treat me so discourteously," goes the old song. Rebuffed as Edmonton's head coach in 2001, Don Matthews had been seething ever since. For Don "Captain Ahab" Matthews, the Eskimos have become his personal Moby Dick. Mike Pringle, rejected in favor of Lawrence Phillips by Matthews in Montreal, was determined to script the final act by playing the starring role. Alouette quarterback Anthony Calvillo wanted post-season respect to go along with his Most Outstanding Player Award. Ricky Ray

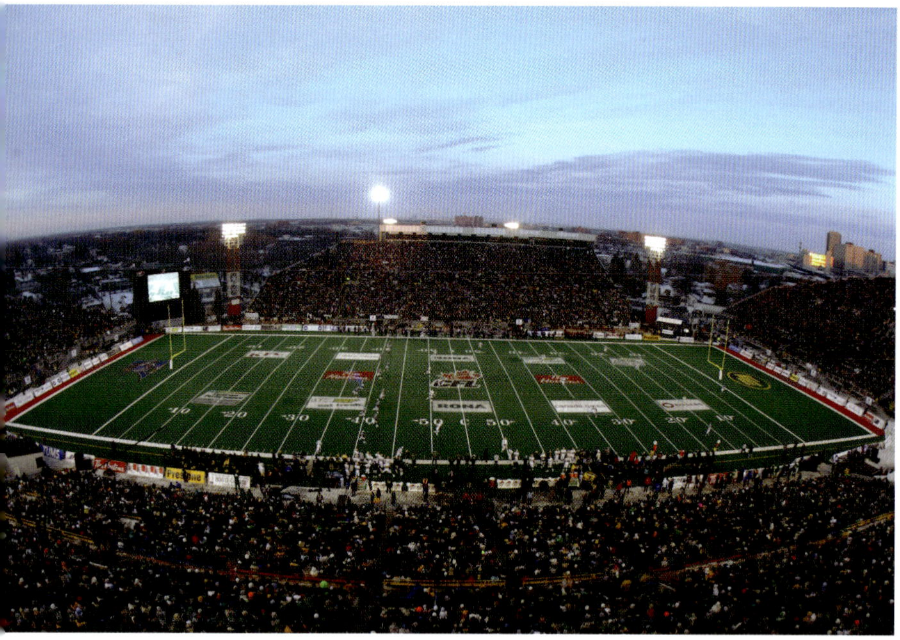

Opening kickoff at Taylor Field, November 16, 2003.

wanted a ring on his resumé before going to the NFL next spring. The personal stakes were high.

It would be Edmonton's outstanding passing attack against Montreal's living on the edge defense comprised of Barron Miles, Reggie Durden, Wayne Shaw, Omar Evans and William Loftus. Because veterans Shaw and Evans hadn't played well in the Eastern final, Matthews opted to bench them in favor of rookies D.J. Johnson and Brandon Williams. Lark linebackers Tim Strickland, Kelvin Johnson, the Eastern nominee for Outstanding Defensive Player, and Duane Butler would back up a tough defensive line featuring Marc Megna, Ed Philion, Adriano Belli and Anwar Stewart.

Edmonton's defense would have to deal with the season's Most Outstanding Player in Anthony Calvillo, the Outstanding Canadian in Ben Cahoon, as well as Jermaine Copeland, Pat Woodcock and Sylvain Girard. Criticized for lack of a running game, Matthews said, "We want our tailback to carry the ball 15 meaningful times a game and gain 80 yards." He settled for 44 yards on nine carries and lost.

Before arriving in Regina, Matthews sent a videotape to the league office that detailed the Eskimo secondary's indiscretions. By doing so, he accused the referees of letting Edmonton get away with murder. This was surprising for a man who practically never reacts to officials in any way. The move would backfire.

The Eskimos' Donny Brady wouldn't take the bait when the media asked him about the accusation of illegal play. "We don't have no reaction," he said emphatically. "We've never seen the video. We think the officials do a good job."

Of course you do. As to the hit he took from Matt Dominguez in the Western final, Brady allowed that, "It felt like I'd made about twenty tackles. He gave me a good shot. I had a little bit of soreness for a couple of days, but I feel fine now." He didn't resent the hit nor would he change his style. "Naw, I'm not going to change my game. I mean, I figure if I'm going to be physical, I have to take a few shots. If I give 'em, I've got to be willing to take 'em."

After Prime Minister-in-Waiting Paul Martin supervised the coin toss, Regina native Matt Kellett kicked off for the Alouettes. Shortly after 5:00 P.M., the temperature was -4°C with the wind out of the southeast at 19 km/hr.

Ricky Ray went after Montreal's defensive back rookies right away. On the fifth play of the game, Ray threw 43 yards to Ed Hervey, who was covered by D.J. Johnson. That made it first and goal from four yards out. Mike Pringle took it the rest of the way. Edmonton 7, Alouettes 0.

"Getting off to a good start like that really pumps a team up," Ray said later. "It set the tone for the game. We wanted to keep them back on their heels and we did."

Edmonton opened the second quarter with a first down on their 40-yard line. Pringle gained two before Ray passed to Troy Mills for 29 yards. The ball at Montreal's 37, Pringle picked up three tough yards. Edmonton was moved back to the 41 on a procedure call. Ray then threw 41 yards to Jason Tucker for a touchdown. Edmonton 14, Montreal 0.

Were the Eskimos picking on the rookie corners? Tucker laughed. "I'm a happy guy, smiling all the time. When I saw two young guys on the corners I smiled a little more and went 'Whoo!' " Tucker had a field day against D.J. Johnson. "He started backing off once I beat him. I noticed that."

Tom Higgins acknowledged it was part of the game plan to exploit the Montreal rookies.

"Absolutely. That's why we went after them right away. We were going to test them, but we knew that our challenge was going to be whether we could afford our quarterback enough time to actually throw the ball to the receivers."

Just when it looked like the rout was on, Anthony Calvillo mounted a 71-yard, six-play drive ending with a sensational individual effort and a bit of razzle-dazzle. Ben Cahoon made the play of the day with a flat-out one-handed catch for a 32-

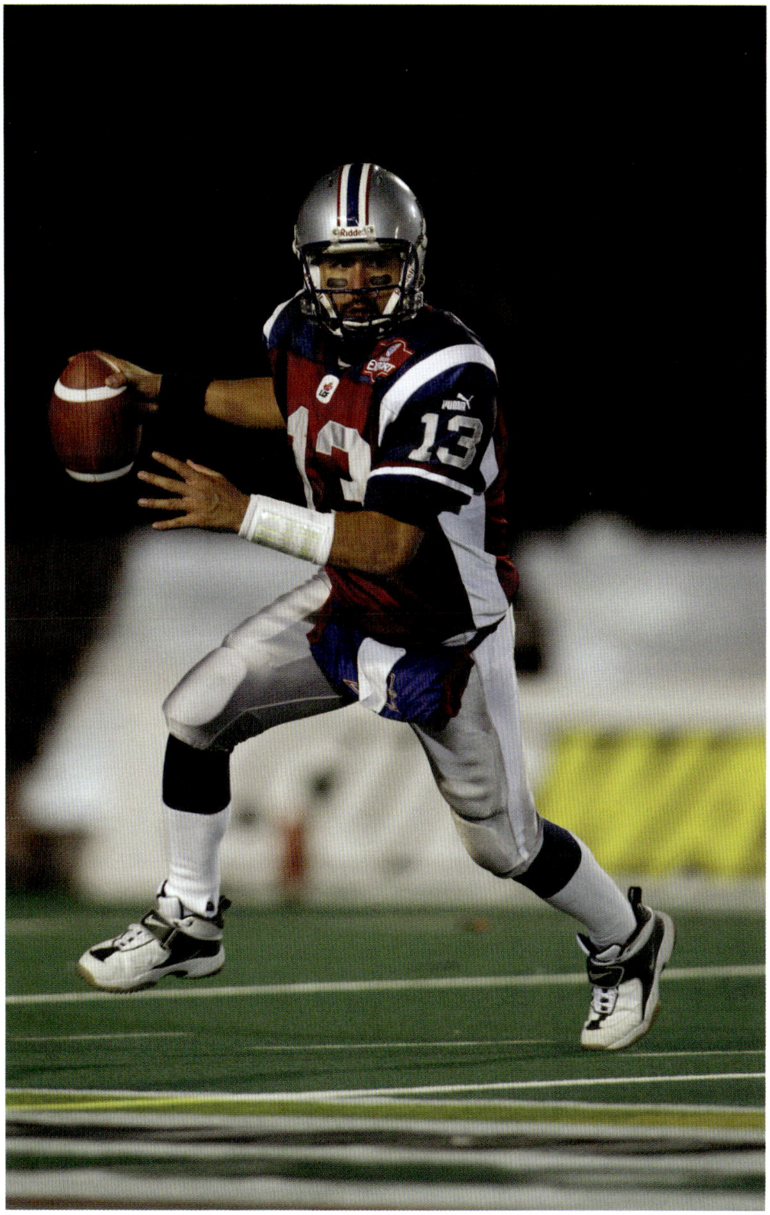

Anthony Calvillo, the CFL's Most Outstanding Player, 2003, on the run in the season finale.

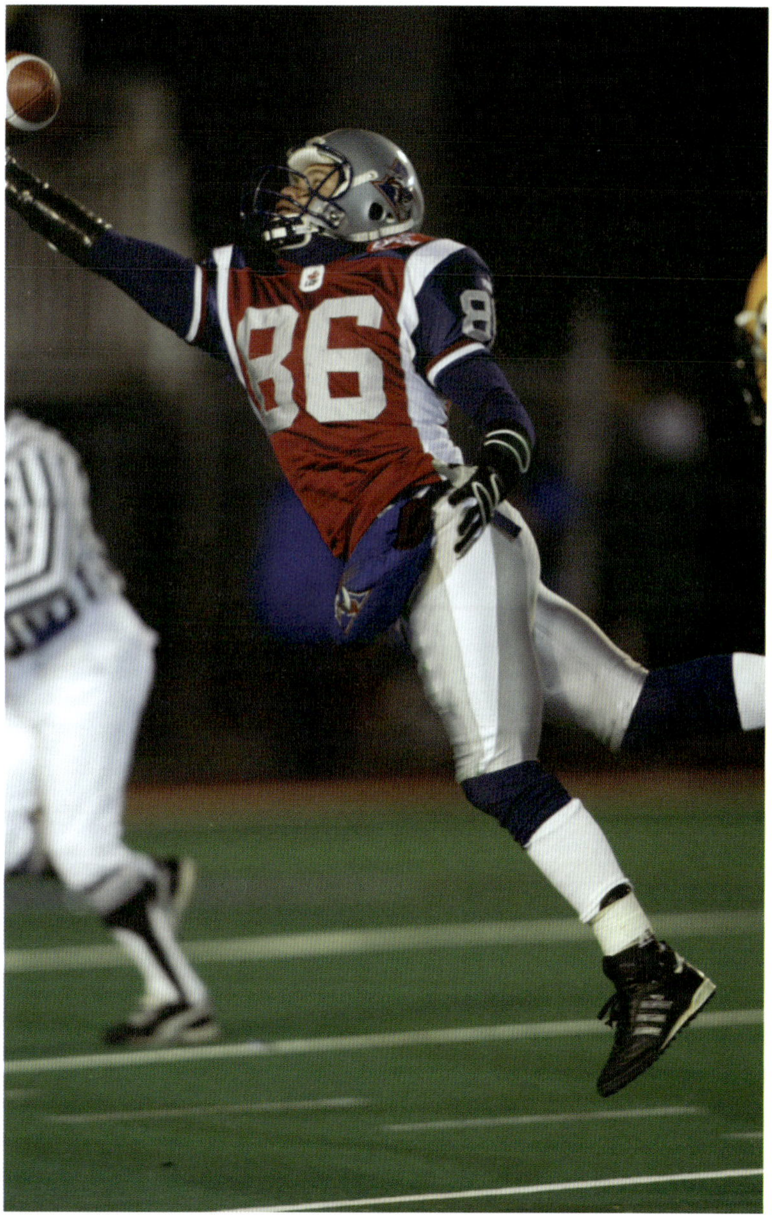

Alouette Ben Cahoon shows why he was named the Outstanding Canadian of 2003 and the Most Valuable Canadian in the Grey Cup.

yard gain that put the ball on the Esks' four-yard line. From there, Calvillo handed off to Whitaker, who threw a pass to the wide-open Pat Woodcock in the end zone. Edmonton led by seven. Three plays later Kevin Johnson recovered a Mike Pringle fumble at the Eskimo 32. Calvillo cashed in on the very next play with a touchdown pass to Sylvain Girard. Tie ball game.

After the kickoff, Edmonton couldn't move the ball, so Sean Fleming had to punt. The usually sure-handed Keith Stokes fumbled the ball on the Montreal 40-yard line. Again Ray took advantage of an opportunity and hooked up with Tucker for another touchdown. Edmonton 21, Montreal 14. That 16-yard strike was set up when Brandon Williams' tight coverage foiled a second down pass to Winston October–only to have the hapless D.J. Johnson called for interference on another receiver.

Continuing the scoring spree, the Alouettes marched 65 yards in five plays with Ben Cahoon hauling in the touchdown pass. Later he would be named Canadian Player of the Game. The score was tied once again.

Edmonton wasn't finished. Forced to punt three plays after the Montreal kickoff, they recovered the ball right back when Stokes coughed it up again, this time into Brady's arms at the Alouette 20. Fleming converted the turnover into a field goal, and Edmonton led Montreal at the half 24–21. The two teams had combined for 38 points in the second quarter.

After enjoying Bryan Adams and the rest of the halftime show, the 50,909 fans in attendance expected more of the same. They didn't get it. After a 15-minute lapse, the Eskimo defense shut the door. All Montreal could manage the rest of the way was a 70-yard Matt Kellett punt single at 9:59 of the third

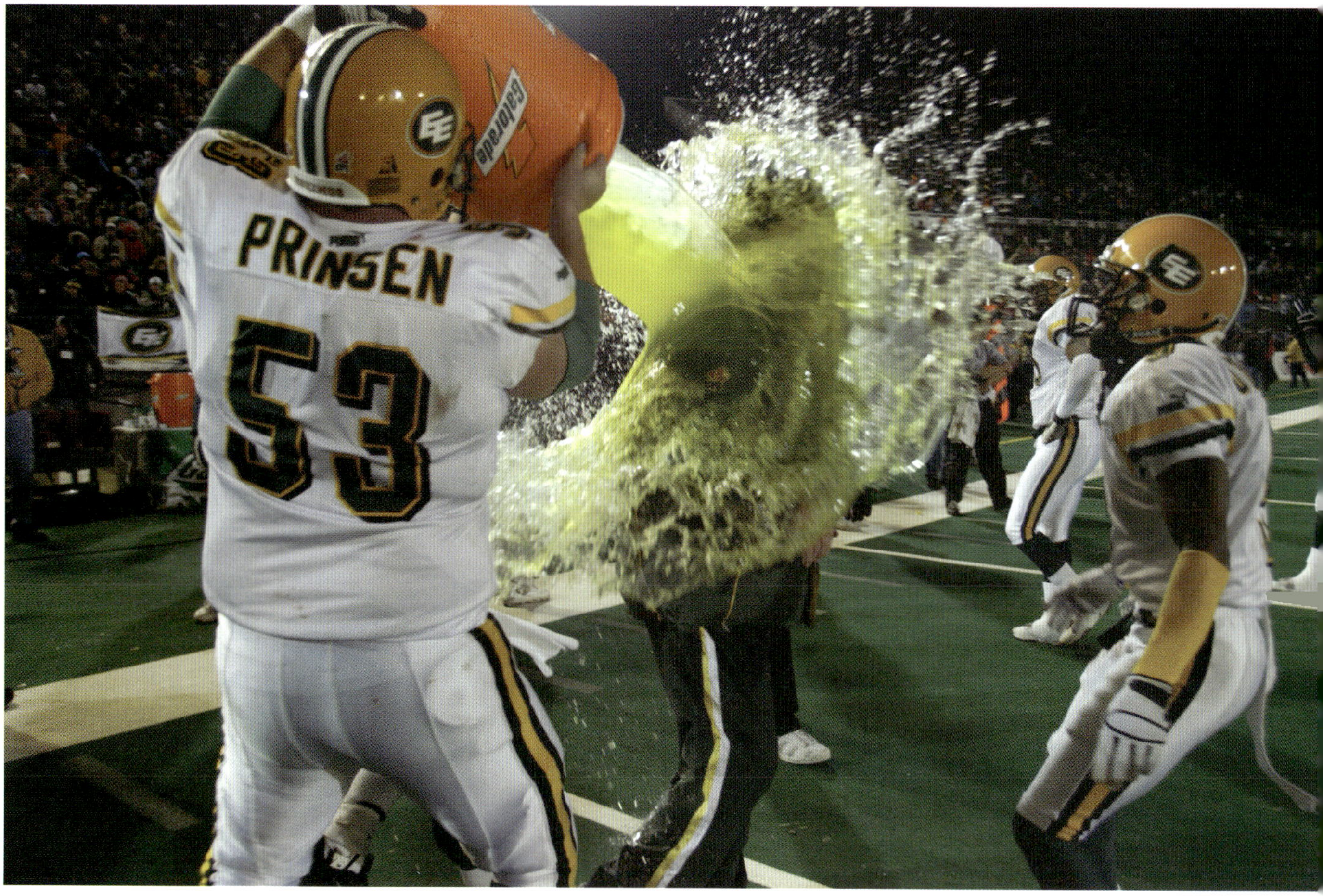

quarter. Finally displaying the killer instinct of a champion, the Eskimos added a Ricky Ray touchdown and Sean Fleming field goal to win 34–22, their 12th Grey Cup and first in ten years.

Commissioner Tom Wright presented the 94-year-old trophy to the 38-year-old offensive lineman Leo Groenewegen.

Later in the locker room, NFL-bound Ricky Ray was asked how he felt.

"It's really hard to explain," he replied. We play the game for this reason. Anytime you set a goal like this and go out and accomplish it, it's an awesome feeling."

The brilliant, young cool-as-a-cucumber quarterback completed 22 of 32 passes for 301 yards and two touchdowns. Eight different players caught passes, including Ed Hervey, who left the game early with a groin pull. Ray acknowledged his talented teammates. "Being on a great team helps a whole lot. Just being in the right place at the right time, coming to an organization that knows how to win has been a big help to me."

Said Tom Higgins, "Every game Ricky played this year, he grew. The expectations were so high. People were thinking that we weren't going to lose any football games, and that's very unreasonable, especially in the West with

Tim Prinsen gives Coach Tom Higgins the traditional Gatorade shower.

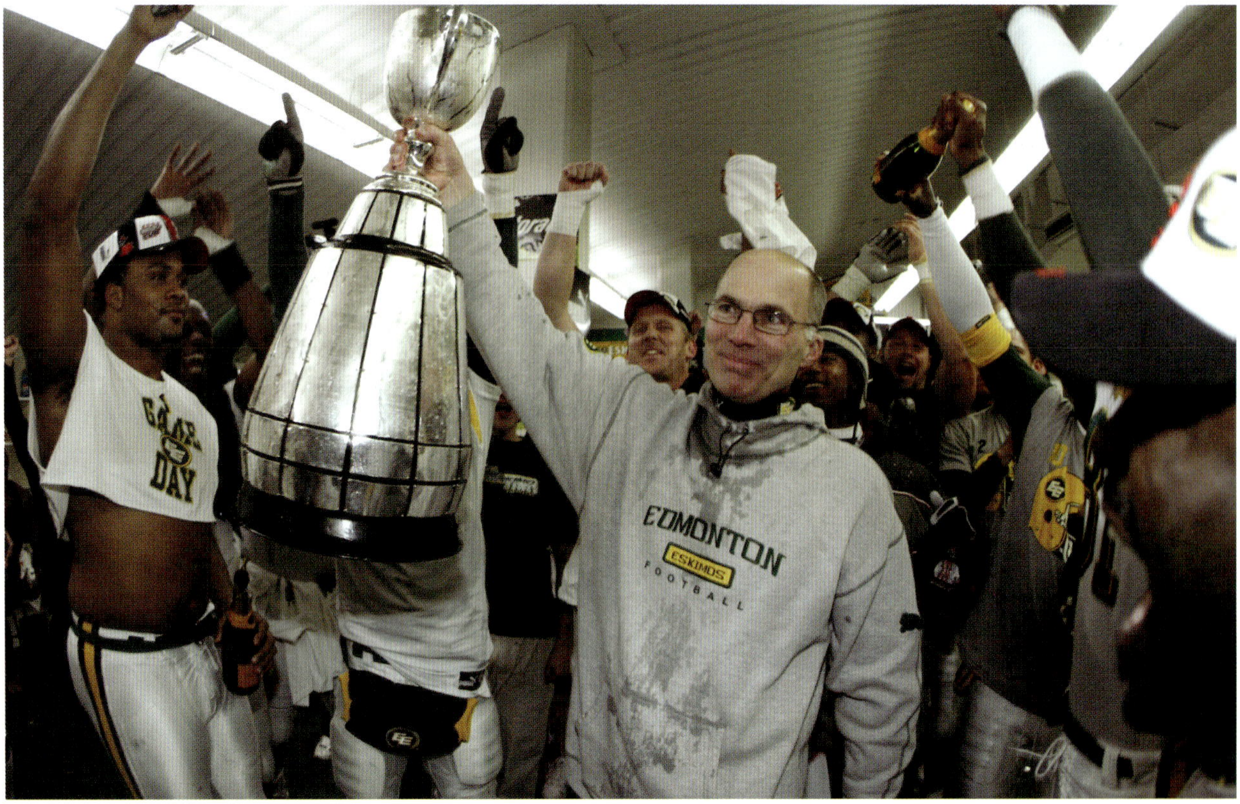

Professor Higgins holds the Cup to the cheers of his players.

such tough opponents. He never lost his poise or his confidence. We grew as Ricky grew. We were able to do things that we weren't able to do last year just because he understood everything that was going on around him. As he improved, so did our offense."

Higgins also spoke of game MVP Jason Tucker. "We missed Ed Hervey. He pulled that groin. He tried to come back but couldn't. We had the ability to move our receivers around. One of the most unselfish players on this team is Jason Tucker because he played in the shadow of Terry Vaughn and Ed Hervey. But we knew when we asked him to make plays, he would do so."

Tucker had seven receptions for 132 yards and two touchdowns–the first time since July 31 in Ottawa that he had been called upon to make more than three catches in a game. He, too, talked only of team. "It's fun playing with my quarterback, Ricky Ray, my offensive line, the whole team. It's been one big team effort all year long. We set out with a big goal, to come and win it this year and not to be denied and that's what we did."

The quarterback agreed. "We had a feeling of loss after last year's Grey Cup game, and we wanted a chance to come back and win it. That was our focus all year long. When we played Montreal in the past we haven't played well together as a team. One of our areas usually had a let down. This year we played solid all across the board, and it wasn't any different tonight."

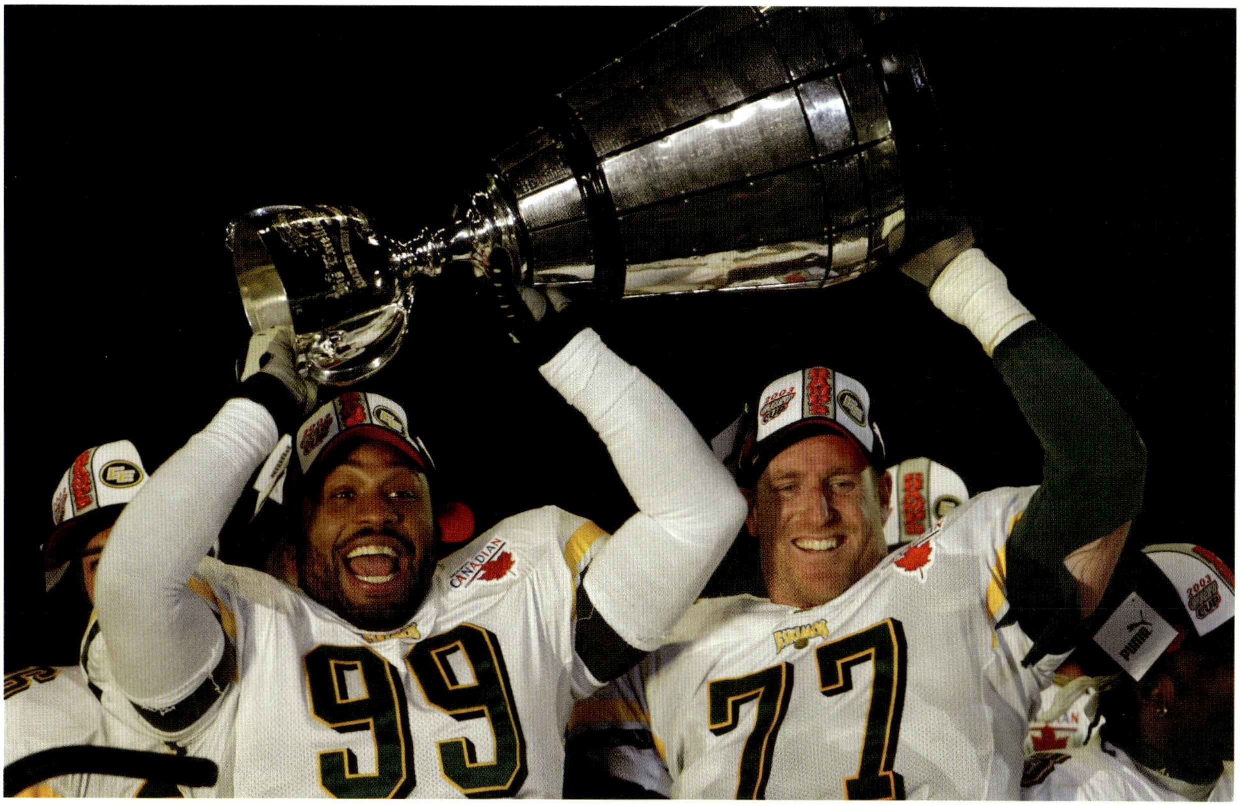

No. 99 Sheldon Benoit and No. 77 A.J. Gass celebrate the Edmonton Eskimos' 12th Grey Cup.

In the 90th Grey Cup in 2002, Edmonton had dominated Montreal but had missed important opportunities and lost. In Grey Cup '91, the Eskimo defense created opportunities that the offense cashed in.

"That is very well put," Higgins agreed. "We felt that the reason the Montreal Alouettes won last year is because they made plays. When we had to make plays in order to win this football game, we were able to do that. We did that early, then they got hot and we were able to shut them down and control the football game in the second half."

"Last year we didn't make the big plays—this year we did," said Ray.

With so much attention lavished on the offense, it would be easy to minimize the contribution of the defense. Coordinator Greg Marshall said, "We got off to a great start and then kind of lost it a bit in the second quarter. But in the second half, we were all over them.

"It wasn't real fancy. Our guys just lined up and got after them. It was a great effort. We talked before the game about it being important that when they had an opportunity to make a play they made it. We had guys taking turns making plays all night."

Don Matthews responded to the criticism of his decision to go with the rookie corners. "It's pretty obvious that penalties and turnovers were the difference—they were all on one side. Our rookie corners were not the reason we lost the football game. We made enough

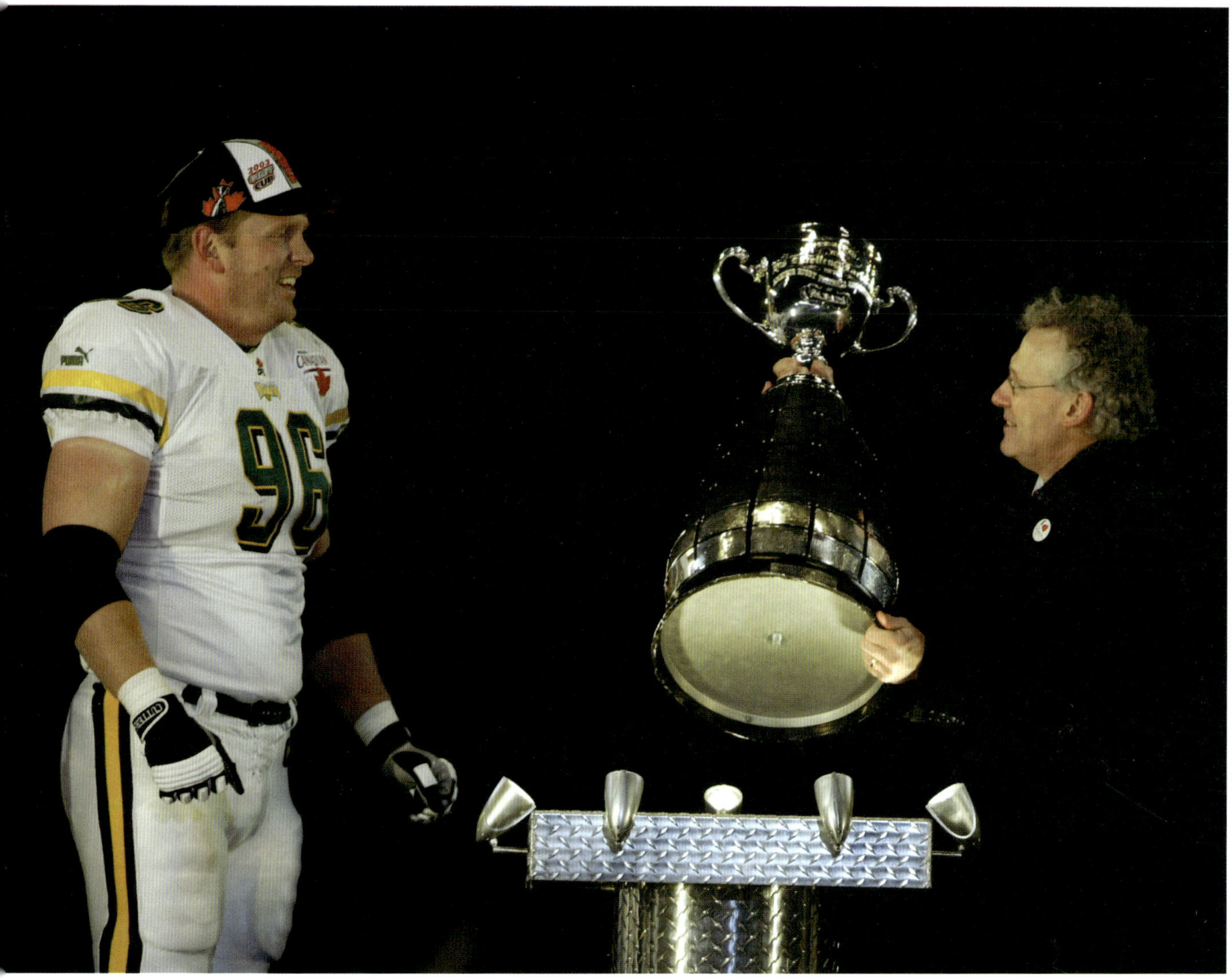

Great veteran Leo Groenewegen accepts the Grey Cup from CFL Commissioner Tom Wright.

mistakes, but I don't care if we had Superman on the field for Tucker's touchdown, that was a perfectly thrown pass that couldn't have been stopped."

So Ned Flanders beat The Don. "It seems true in the CFL that you have to lose before you can win," Higgins said. "What gave us confidence was the fact that the whole year there was a resolve. It started the day after last year's Grey Cup. The players wanted the opportunity to do it all over again. They made sacrifices during the off-season. We had a little adversity early on that I think helped refocus us on the direction we wanted to go. I really couldn't be happier for the Edmonton Eskimo organization. It seems like it has been a long drought, but we've still been proud in all the years because we've always been competitive, we've always given our best effort. But now it doesn't get any sweeter than when you finally win the last game of the year."

Edmonton, Alberta. City of Champions once again.